AUDIOLOGICAL EVALUATION
OF THE
PEDIATRIC PATIENT

Publication Number 570

AMERICAN LECTURE SERIES®

A Monograph in

AMERICAN LECTURES IN SPEECH AND HEARING

Edited by

ROBERT WEST, *Director*

Speech and Hearing Center

Brooklyn College

Brooklyn, New York

Second Printing

Audiological Evaluation of the Pediatric Patient

By

MAURICE H. MILLER, Ph.D.
Assistant Professor, Division of Otolaryngology
State University of New York, Downstate Medical Center
Brooklyn, New York
Coordinator, Hearing and Speech Clinic
Kings County Hospital Center
Brooklyn, New York
Audiological Consultant, Bureau for Handicapped Children
New York, New York

and

IRA A. POLISAR, M.D., F.A.C.S.
Associate Professor and Head, Division of Otolaryngology
State University of New York, Downstate Medical Center
Brooklyn, New York
Director, Otolaryngology Service
Kings County Hospital Center
Brooklyn, New York
Director, Department of Otolaryngology
Long Island College Hospital
Brooklyn, New York

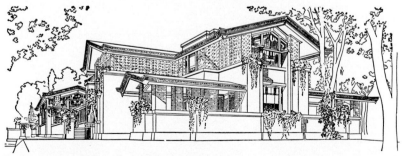

CHARLES   C   THOMAS   •   PUBLISHER
Springfield   •   Illinois   •   U. S. A.

Published and Distributed Throughout the World by
CHARLES C THOMAS • PUBLISHER
BANNERSTONE HOUSE
301-327 East Lawrence Avenue, Springfield, Illinois, U.S.A.
NATCHEZ PLANTATION HOUSE
735 North Atlantic Boulevard, Fort Lauderdale, Florida, U.S.A.

First Printing, 1964
Second Printing, 1971

*With THOMAS BOOKS careful attention is given to all details of
manufacturing and design. It is the Publisher's desire to present books
that are satisfactory as to their physical qualities and artistic possibilities
and appropriate for their particular use. THOMAS BOOKS will be true
to those laws of quality that assure a good name and good will.*

Printed in the United States of America
00-2

DEDICATION

To my wife, Anita,

for her constant encouragement from "start to finish" and her relentless but necessary insistence that this book be finally completed

M.H.M.

To "Liz"

and our three wonderful sons, Joseph, Stephen and Roger

I.A.P.

FOREWORD

ONE TERM THAT is found with increasing frequency in our literature on health sciences is *paramedical*. To some this means *quasimedical*. But more and more it is coming to designate that which is truly medical, but that which the medical colleges of our educational establishment do not include in their curricula. The paramedical specialty of *audiology* is based upon a broad foundation, including those aspects of conventional medicine that are concerned with diseases of the ear and the auditory tracts, plus aspects of the sciences and arts of electronics, acoustics, education, psychology, and speech pathology. Audiology is a highly technical profession requiring a rich background of training and experience.

The dignity of this paramedical specialty is distinctly enhanced by the works and writings of Drs. Miller and Polisar. They have here written a document so scholarly that it may well rank with the best handbooks in conventional medical literature. In special terms this book could well be labeled *Pediatric Audiology*. The authors are well qualified to write a text in the areas that are implied by this dual title; and they have clearly done so.

ROBERT WEST, *Editor*

PREFACE

THE IMPETUS FOR the establishment of major audiological diagnostic facilities in medical institutions usually orignates with a physician, typically a pediatrician or an otolaryngologist who recognizes the need for such services in his community. The authors believe that much of the material contained in this manual will be of value to such physicians in the organization and conduct of these services. It is also hoped that general practitioners, pediatricians and internists who typically are the first professional persons to encounter children with speech and hearing problems will read these pages and recognize the need for *early* referral of these children to properly equipped and manned diagnostic facilities. Speech and hearing therapists, educators of the deaf, clinical psychologists, nurses and other personnel who encounter children with definite or suspected speech and hearing disorders may also profit from the information contained herein.

The far-reaching repercussions of delay in diagnosis has been cogently brought to the attention of the professional and lay public in such areas as cancer and heart disease. The necessity of extending this warning to the early identification and diagnosis of disorders of communication is apparent to the authors who are asked daily to work with children who required attention years before. The secondary psychological problems which too frequently result from failure to administer appropriate treatment in time are often as difficult to handle as the basic problem. The loss of time further deprives the youngster of the additional years of rehabilitation and special education which he often requires if he is to function successfully with his non-handicapped contemporaries.

The authors wish to express their sincere appreciation to Dr. Robert W. West for his initial suggestions regarding the preparation of this text and his invaluable assistance and suggestions freely offered at all stages of this work. We are further indebted to the following persons for their assistance: Mrs. Donrue C. Poole, Pediatric Audiologist in the Hearing and Speech Clinic of Kings County Hospital Center for case material included in Chapter V., Mrs. Betty Schwartz for final corrections and typing of the manuscript, Mrs. Elizabeth Cuzzort, Director of the Medical Illustrations Department and her staff for assistance in the preparation of the illustrations and audiograms and Mrs. Helen Kovaks, Head Librarian and Miss Elizabeth L. Keenan, Senior Librarian at the Medical Library of the State University of New York Downstate Medical Center for assistance in preparation of the references for this text. Finally, our appreciation is extended to our teachers, colleagues, students and patients for all they have contributed to our understanding of the infinite complexities of communication disorders.

MAURICE H. MILLER
IRA A. POLISAR

CONTENTS

AUDIOLOGICAL EVALUATION
OF THE
PEDIATRIC PATIENT

Chapter I

INTRODUCTION AND CLASSIFICATION

INTRODUCTION

THE EVALUATION of the hearing of young children is a highly specialized area, and a challenging problem, of clinical audiology. Many of the techniques used in hearing measurement of adults are not applicable to young children, particularly those with retarded *speech* and *language* development. Problems of hearing evaluation are complicated by the presence of pathological entities, other than reduced hearing sensitivity on a peripheral basis, which may contribute significantly to the child's communication disorder. Such problems include central nervous system disorders, mental retardation and different degrees of emotional disturbance. Frequently, more than one of these factors coexist and contribute to the problem of hearing evaluation.

Such children require, during the course of diagnostic workup, a more or less comprehensive evaluation of their hearing. These children also show lack of, or inconsistent response to, auditory stimuli and must be clearly differentiated from children with true hearing losses. The presenting complaints to the family physician are usually identical for all these children, namely delayed speech development and/or lack of response to sound.

The pediatric population undergoing evaluation in audiology centers is characterized, to an increasing degree, by children with multiple problems contributing to their communication disorders. This change in patient population is at least partly a reflection of the improved obstetrical care now available in our medical institutions which is resulting in the salvage of many lives which previously had been lost. The developments responsible for the increased number of survivors include the use of exchange transfusions for offspring of parents with Rh and other blood incompatibilities, recognition of the relationship of oxygen deprivation to irreversible brain damage in infants, improved techniques in operative delivery, and recognition of the relationship between rubella in the first trimester of pregnancy and the triad of congenital cataracts, sensorineural hearing loss and cardiac defects. These developments, while saving lives, have complicated the already difficult problems of evaluation and rehabilitation of children with auditory pathology.

The population in schools for the deaf includes fewer children with "simple" peripheral reduction in auditory sensitivity and greater numbers of aphasic and "aphasoid" children, autistic and schizophrenic children, children with mental retardation and "central" hearing impairments secondary to diffuse brain damage as well as combinations of these and other auditory pathology. It has been conservatively estimated that a minimum of 1,500 speech and hearing clinicians must be trained each year to meet the needs of the nearly 9,000,000 Americans with speech and hearing problems. At the present time, only 400 therapists are being trained in the speech and hearing field each year. (1)

The changing nature of our clinic population makes increasing demands on our already understaffed facilities and emphasizes the necessity for the development of adequate diagnostic and therapeutic services for our patients as well as appropriate educational facilities for handling children with problems heretofore unrecognized.

Children with cerebral palsy, particularly of the athethoid type, often have high frequency sensorineural hearing losses affecting speech perception and production. Unilateral and bilateral sensorineural hearing losses are a not infrequent accompaniment of some of the exanthematous diseases, particularly measles and mumps. Children with cleft palates show a high incidence of conductive losses which may contribute significantly to problems in rehabilitation. These examples are illustrative of the many conditions reaching the attention of the family physician in which hearing disorders often occur and which require adequate evaluation and management.

Some audiologists, who do well in evaluating and rehabilitating hard-of-hearing adults, experience considerable difficulty and insecurity in working with a hard-of-hearing child. The term "Paedo-audiology" (2) has been suggested to designate the area of audiology involving the auditory assessment and rehabilitation of children.

CLASSIFICATION

There is considerable confusion regarding appropriate terms to designate different types of auditory pathology in children. The term auditory pathology is used to designate all forms of communication disorders in children rather than limiting its use to children having reduced auditory sensitivity secondary to peripheral impairment. At least some of the differences of opinion among workers in this area appear to involve primarily semantic problems which have not as yet been resolved. For example, some specialists refuse to use the term "aphasia" to apply to central language problems in children (3) while others consider the term appropriate and useful regardless of the age group for which it is employed (4). The designation "central hearing impairment" or central deafness continues to be a highly nebulous term defined differently by different authorities, a difficulty which probably reflects our present limited knowledge of the physiology and pathology of the higher central auditory pathways and their relation to specific clinical entities.

Many systems of classification have been suggested by other authors. None of these has been universally accepted. This is because of an inherent problem of crossing anatomical and functional terminology within the classification and because of limited knowledge as to the physiology and pathology of central auditory structures. For purpose of this text, we outline below our classification knowing that it has its limitations but attempting to reduce them by the inclusion of definitions within the text.

CLASSIFICATION OF AUDITORY PATHOLOGY

I. Reduced Hearing Sensitivity Due to *Peripheral Lesions*
    A. Conductive
    B. Sensorineural (Cochlear)
II. Reduced Hearing Sensitivity Due to *Retrocochlear Lesions*
    A. Sensorineural (Retrocochlear)
    B. Central
III. Central Language Disorders

IV.   Other Etiological Factors Related to Speech and Language Disturbance
    A.   Emotional
    B.   Intellectual

It should be noted that the term sensorineural hearing loss is included under Peripheral as well as Non-Peripheral categories of reduced hearing sensitivity because such losses may have their anatomical locus in the cochlea as well as in structures medial to the cochlea. We are, therefore, dealing with the problem of trying to identify in one classification: (a) types of hearing loss, and (b) anatomical location. It should be borne in mind that a sensorineural lesion will appear under Category I (Reduced Hearing Sensitivity Due to Peripheral Lesions) when it is cochlear in origin and under Category II (Reduced Hearing Sensitivity Due to Retrocochlear Lesions) when retrocochlear structures are involved.

I.   Reduced Hearing Sensitivity Due to Peripheral Lesions

A.   Conductive Losses of Hearing

These impairments result from abnormality of the external and middle ear and are particularly significant in children because of the frequent occurrence of this kind of pathology and the possibility of their medical or surgical correction. The most frequent cause of conductive impairment in children is some form of otitis media which is a common complication of upper respiratory infections. Serous and purulent middle ear effusions, hypertrophied lymphoid tissue in the oro- and naso-pharynx, and retracted, scarred and perforated tympanic membranes are among the otological findings in children with conductive losses of hearing. Audiometrically, conductive impairments affect hearing via air conduction by varying degrees depending on the nature and severity of the pathology. However, conductive impairments generally do not exceed a maximum air conduction loss of 60-65 db. The configuration of the air conduction curve will depend upon whether the pathology alters the conductive mechanism as to its stiffness, mass, and/or resistance. (5)

Bone conduction in cases of conductive hearing impairment is classically within normal limits, or it may be better than normal. The phenomenon of hypersensitive bone conduction in cases of conductive hearing loss is believed by some to be associated with the failure of bone conducted sounds to be masked by ambient room noise as occurs in persons with non-conductive impairments. In some cases, particularly when the pathology affects the mobility of the stapes and round window membrane, bone, as well as air conduction sensitivity may be affected by middle ear disease. Palva and Ojala (6) reported that in nearly one-third of cases with simple acute otitis media, bone conduction is abnormally poor until healing of the middle ear occurs.

In serous or adhesive otitis media, patients may show a curve typical of sensorineural loss of hearing with some impairment of bone conduction primarily affecting the higher frequencies. The reason for this is either serous secretions which fill the window niches of the middle ear or adhesions and thickened membranes which impair mobility of both windows. In the absence of inflammation, both air and bone conduction instantly return to normal values when the serous fluid is aspirated. Such bone conduction losses which are secondary to "impedance" factors do not reflect true neural degeneration and may be reversible by appropriate otological procedures, such as myringotomy, paracentesis or inflation of the Eustachian tube. An increasing number of otologists and audiologists are reporting clinical findings indicating that bone conduction sensitivity is affected by factors other than neural degeneration in cases of otosclerosis and otitis media. (7, 8, 9)

B. Sensorineural Losses of Hearing (Cochlear)

Peripheral sensorineural losses involve destruction or damage to the inner or outer hair cells along the basilar membrane of the cochlea, or pathology affecting the fluid system of the inner ear. There is no otological evidence of these conditions from the physical examination of the patient and diagnosis involves the use of various functional tests of hearing and other procedures, such as vestibular and neurological examinations, and x-ray studies. Audiometric tests classically show an equal loss of hearing for air- and bone-conducted sounds in this instance. Such losses frequently affect high frequencies to a greater degree than the low frequency portion of the hearing range. However, it should be noted that sensorineural losses may be associated with a flat audiometric configuration, a "saucer" shaped audiogram or a rising contour.

Sensorineural losses of the cochlear type are typically accompanied by the "recruitment" phenomenon which refers to an abnormal increase in the loudness sensation of a tone as its intensity is increased above the pathological threshold. These losses are sometimes genetically transmitted although they are more frequently associated with adventitious etiologies such as the effects of ototoxic drugs (e.g., dihydrostreptomycin, neomycin and kanamycin) or diseases such as encephalitis, meningitis and measles.

II.   Reduced Hearing Sensitivity Due to Retrocochlear Lesions

A. Retrocochlear lesions refer to conditions affecting structures centrad to the cochlea. Spiral ganglion pathology or the various forms of eighth nerve degeneration fall into this category. Such pathology is not frequently encountered in children except for uncontrolled suppurative infections of the middle ear which, in the pre-antibiotic era, not infrequently invaded the bony and membranous labyrinth and even the dura producing destruction of cochlear neural structures and meningitic involvement. (10) In adults, hearing loss secondary to acoustic neuromata, cerebello-pontine angle tumors and von Recklinghausen's neurofibromas would fall under this classification. The first two of these conditions are usually unilateral and typically characterized by the absence of the recruitment phenomenon.

B. The terms "central deafness" and "central hearing impairment" are used by the authors to refer to reduction in hearing sensitivity due to lesions within the central nervous system. The dorsal and ventral cochlear nuclei may be considered as the boundary between the peripheral and central portions of the auditory transmissive system. Damage to the cochlear nuclei or structures centrad to them including areas of the temporal cortex concerned with primary auditory reception would fall into the classification of central deafness as defined herein.

The behavioral and audiometric characteristics of children with central hearing impairments have not yet been clearly identified and

described. Clinically, these children are extremely difficult to condition by either subjective or electrophysiological audiometry and
give erratic, bizarre audiometric reponses even after a series of test
sessions.

Tobey (11) believes that lesions of the medial geniculate body
or of the auditory cortex do not result in hearing loss unless they are
bilateral. A number of workers believe that damage on the cortical
level alone produces no reduction in hearing sensitivity and that such
pathology becomes evident through tests which explore more sensi-
tive and subtle dimensions than pure tone and speech reception thresholds. J. Matzker, (12) for example, considers auditory localization
a purely cerebral function and has suggested a series of special tests
which he considers valuable in the diagnosis of central disturbances.
In his tonal test, short bursts of tone of equal intensity and with a
small and variable alteration in time of arrival strike both ears. Lateralization was found to be optimal at an interval of 0.633 msec. between the two sounds; shorter differences provoke impressions which
correspond proportionally to a less lateralized or nonlateralized perception. There is a median zone called the median band in which
lateralization does not occur. This band increases with age and
reaches its greatest band width in the geriatric population. An auditory disturbance of cerebral origin is assumed in cases of deviation
of the median band without a difference in auditory thresholds of
the two ears. A deviation toward the right side suggests a lesion in
the left hemisphere or in the posterior right fossa, and vice versa.
In the presence of extensive cerebral processes the deviation depends
on the inferior extension of the lesion; e.g., a tumor of the left hemisphere reaching the left posterior fossa will be revealed by a deviation of the median band toward the left side in the same manner
as a more limited process of the right hemisphere. Matzker's tests
appear quite promising but require a number of modifications to
eliminate the test artifacts which result from limitations of some of
his instrumentation. Several changes in test methodology are also
required. Further development of his approach to the diagnosis of
central lesions is currently in progress at the Audiology Research
Laboratory of Long Island College Hospital in Brooklyn, New York,
made possible by a research grant from the Vocational Rehabilitation Administration.

Jerger (13) believes that discrimination tests as conventionally performed fail to reveal any deviation from normal findings in cases of cortical involvement. However, phonetically balanced words presented through a low pass filter or at low sensation levels will frequently reveal discrimination scores considerably below those obtained with normal subjects in the ear contralateral to the lesion. The observation by Proctor, Gurdjian and Webster, (14) in 1956, that the clinical and pathological evidence of true central deafness is inconclusive remains largely true at the present time although much valuable information has been added to our understanding of these challenging problems.

Children with damage to central auditory pathways are encountered clinically although specialists in the field are unable to agree on the basis of this diagnosis and much remains to be learned about the audiological and other characteristics of these children. Educational and therapeutic procedures for handling the communicative problems resulting from these conditions are receiving increased attention. Much additional investigation into all phases of this difficult problem is necessary.

III.   Central Language Disorders

It is now recognized that speech and language retardation in some children is related to an inability to comprehend and/or utilize language because of certain central nervous system deficits. Infantile or childhood aphasia, oligophasia, central auditory imperception and auditory agnosia are some of the terms which have been used to designate this condition. The term aphasia is used to designate impairment affecting the use of language symbols; the apraxias and dysarthrias are not included since these terms refer to sub-symbolic speech functions. Many, and according to some a majority, of these children show no abnormal results on standard neurological test procedures including electroencephalography. Rapin, (15) for example, found that of a group of twenty-six children with communication disorders attending a school for the deaf, none showed significant findings on a standard neurological examination and only one showed abnormal EEG findings. Thirteen children in this group had previously been diagnosed as "dysacusis with or without demonstrable neurological disturbance."

The diagnosis of aphasia in children is based primarily upon behavioral and developmental characteristics which have been described in detail by Strauss and Lehtinen, (16) Myklebust, (17) and others. Myklebust (18) classifies the etiology of aphasia in children into: 1. Agenesis, or deviations in brain development from the time of conception; and 2. Damage due to trauma occurring after conception. The most frequently found causative factors in the history of aphasic children are anoxia, Rh incompatability, rubella, cerebral hemorrhage occurring at the time of birth, and diseases such as meningitis and encephalitis.

The present authors prefer not to use the term "dysacusis" since it encompasses too great a variety of auditory disturbances. Literally, it refers to a disturbance or aberration in hearing and has already been defined differently in a number of recent texts. Goodhill, (19) for example, suggests that dysacusis can be used as a general heading for a variety of central communication defects including aphasia, psychogenic and hysterical deafness. Davis and Silverman, (20) appear to accept Goodhill's definition of this term but would also include any auditory disturbance not lending itself to correction by simple amplification and therefore, not measurable in decibels. The causes of dysacusis include, according to Davis and Silverman, malformation or injury of either the central nervous system, the auditory nerve, or the auditory sense organ, and include such phenomena as recruitment, diplacusis and discrimination loss. Any or all of the auditory phenomena mentioned can and often do occur with cochlear pathology as, for example, in Ménière's disease. This definition of dysacusis thus includes virtually any non-conductive auditory pathology. This all-inclusive use of the term does not, in our judgment, contribute to a satisfactory classification of auditory pathology in children.

IV. Other Etiological Factors Related to Speech and Language Disturbances

The differential diagnosis of communication disorders in children must include appropriate tests for the evaluation of the intellectual level and emotional status of the child. These areas may contribute significantly to the failure of a child to respond to auditory stimuli and to develop adequate speech and language.

Emotional disturbances present in children with communication disorders may range from relatively mild problems secondary to a peripheral loss of hearing, at one end, to childhood psychosis including autism and schizophrenia, at the other. The services of properly trained psychologists and psychiatrists are a necessary part of the "team approach" to the total evaluation of children with communication disorders. Standardized psychometric and personality inventories are often inappropriate to a population of children with retarded speech and language and must be modified. In some cases, new test batteries must be devised appropriate to the particular population studied. Pediatric neurologists and pediatric psychiatrists whose services are often available in major medical centers, particularly those affiliated with teaching institutions, also contribute significantly to both evaluation and therapy.

Young children whose speech and language deficits are due to severe emotional disorders or intellectual retardation may present clinical pictures similar in many respects to that of children with hearing losses, and the presenting complaints by the parent to the family physician are often similar or identical. Furthermore, as mentioned earlier, more than one of these factors often coexist and these contributory factors must be identified as clearly as possible with existing techniques so that appropriate medical, surgical and rehabilitative procedures may be planned and carried out.

In this text, only the audiological evaluation of the child with communication disorders will be considered. The evaluation of the hearing of the child represents only one phase of the total diagnostic study which children with communication disorders require. No one specialist is equipped to provide all of the diagnostic services indicated, but each should have working knowledge and appreciation of the contributions of other disciplines, medical and non-medical. This type of multifaceted evaluation is best provided by the facilities available in a medical setting where the services of the required specialists are available and can be coordinated into a functioning "team."

REFERENCES

(1) ASHA Committee on Legislation: The need for adequately trained

speech pathologists and audiologists. Asha, *1*:138, (Dec.) 1959.

(2) Huizing, H. C.: Paedo-audiology, its present status and future development, in *Proceedings of the International Course in Paedo-Audiology*. Groningen University, The Netherlands, 1953.

(3) Kastein, S. and Fowler, E. P., Jr.: Differential diagnosis of communication disorders in children referred for hearing tests. *A.M.A. Arch. Otolaryng., 60*:468, 1954.

(4) Myklebust, H. R.: Aphasia in children - diagnosis and training, in Travis, L. E.: *Handbook of Speech Pathology*. Appleton-Century-Crofts, New York, 1957, chap. XIV.

(5) Johansen, H.: Relation of audiograms to the impedance formula. *Acta. Otolaryng.*, supp. *74*:65, 1948.

(6) Palva, T. and Ojala, L.: Middle ear conduction deafness and bone conduction. *Acta. Otolaryng., 45*:137, 1955.

(7) McConnell, F. and Carhart, R.: Influence of fenestration surgery on bone conduction measurements. *Laryngoscope, 62*:1267, (Dec.) 1952.

(8) Kalmon, M., Miller, M. H. and Fowler, E. P., Jr.: Marked improvement in bone conduction. *Ann. Otol. Rhin. & Laryng., 66*:981, (Dec.) 1957.

(9) Sellers, L. M.: False positive perception deafness tests. *Laryngoscope, 69*:493, (May) 1959.

(10) Fowler, E. P.: Diseases of the neural mechanism of hearing: cochlea, auditory nerve and its centers in the medulla and cortex, in Fowler, E. P., Jr., ed: *Loose-Leaf Medicine of the Ear*. Nelson, New York, 1947, chap. VIII, p. 288.

(11) Tobey, H. F.: Symposium: neural mechanism of hearing, V: Etiological and clinical types of so-called "nerve deafness." *Laryngoscope, 47*:598, (Aug.) 1937.

(12) Matzker, J.: The value of the examination of acoustic localization for the diagnosis of cerebral processes. *Ann. Otolaryng., 78*:572, 1961.

(13) Jerger, J.: Medical Audiology Workshop. Estes Park, Colorado, July 29-Aug. 3, 1962.

(14) Proctor, B., Gurdjian, E. S. and Webster, J. E.: The ear in head trauma. *Laryngoscope, 66*:16, (Jan.) 1956.

(15) Rapin, I.: The neurological examination in the diagnosis of communication disorders, part II, pp. 36-38, in *A Differential Study*

of Communication Disorders in a School for the Deaf. Doug-
las, F. M., Fowler, E. P., Jr. and Ryan, G. M.: Project Report
from St. Joseph's School for the Deaf and The Lester A. Hof-
heimer Speech and Hearing Clinic of the Department of Otolaryngology, Columbia Presbyterian Medical Center, New York,
May, 1961.

(16) Strauss, A. A. and Lehtinen, L. E.: *Psychopathology and Education of the Brain-Injured Child.* Grune and Stratton, New York,
1954.

(17) Myklebust, H. R.: *Auditory Disorders in Children:* A Manual for
Differential Diagnosis. Grune and Stratton, New York, 1954.

(18) Myklebust, H. R.: Therapy of aphasia in children, in Travis, L. E.:
Handbook of Speech Pathology. Appleton-Century-Crofts, New
York, 1957, pp. 521-522.

(19) Goodhill, V. P.: Etiology and therapy of deafness, in Travis, L. E.:
Handbook of Speech Pathology. Appleton-Century-Crofts, New
York, 1957, p. 314.

(20) Davis, H. and Silverman, S. R.: *Hearing and Deafness.* Rev. ed.,
Holt, Rinehart and Winston, New York, 1960, p. 555.

Chapter II

GROSS RESPONSES TO UNCALIBRATED
SOUND SOURCES

STANDARD TECHNIQUES of hearing evaluation are not applicable to the very young child who is unable to give a voluntary response to auditory stimuli. In certain infants and young children, the physician or parent may suspect the existence of a hearing loss particularly in those cases in which the history includes a condition often associated with reduced hearing sensitivity. Among such conditions are Rh and other blood incompatibilities, rubella in the first trimester of pregnancy, cerebral hypoxia at or near birth and congenital, familial sensorineural hearing impairments.

The appropriate management of these children depends upon the early detection and proper diagnosis of the auditory problem. Since, as previously noted, conventional techniques are inapplicable at this age, one must rely on *gross responses to uncalibrated sound sources*. Such techniques are frequently employed by physicians as a preliminary screening device in an effort to determine which youngsters require a more comprehensive and detailed evaluation at a specialized center.

GROSS RESPONSES

A.   Palpebral Reflex

One of the best known of these reponses is the acoustico-palpebral reflex which consists of a quick closing and opening movement of the eyelids immediately after an acoustic stimulation of short duration and high intensity. (1) The use of the palpebral reflex for the diagnosis of organic deafness was suggested by Bechterew who found the reflex absent in deaf persons. In performing this proce-

[15]

dure it is important to avoid the simultaneous occurrence of the normal lid movements with the acoustic lid reflex. The eyes must be kept as quiet as possible and the facial muscles relaxed. A child should not be tested while crying. Hahlbrock elicited reflex movements most commonly at 110 db. Since the palpebral reflex occurs only at intense levels of stimulation this procedure has limited value as a quantitative test of hearing function. As with other similar procedures this test, at best, gives information only on whether hearing is present or absent, a finding which can generally be determined with considerable certainty from a careful history based upon an interview with the child's parents.

Froeschels (2) recommends the use of "direct tone introduction" to evaluate the eye muscle reflex. A rubber tube to which an ear olive is attached is inserted into the external auditory meatus, while the other end of the tube touches the opening of a whistle through which the tone is introduced. The procedure involves the use of a set of whistles from Urbantschitsch's organon, comprising a tonal range from about 37 to 716 cycles per second (cps). The reflexes expected as a positive answer to the direct introduction of a tone are blinking, grimaces and, incidentally, the "eye muscle reflex." Froeschels recognizes that the child may respond to the overtones rather than the single notes of a particular whistle. He feels, however, that if there is a positive reaction to different whistles the examiner can safely assume that different tones have been heard since different pipes comprise different overtones and some do not contain any of the overtones appearing in others. A positive response to almost all or to all of the whistles is assumed to indicate the presence of hearing throughout the entire range encompassed by the whistles. The intensity of the different whistles is not specified by Froeschels in his description of this procedure.

B. Startle Reactions

Some examiners, in the initial stages of the hearing evaluation, expose the young child to sounds of increasing intensity until some observable reaction is elicited. The nature of this reaction may be a startle response, such as crying, cessation of play activity, or turning of the head toward the source of sound. This type of procedure may be performed in an ordinary room or office or in a sound field using a calibrated microphone circuit whose output is fed through one or more loudspeakers. A variety of sound stimuli may be employed including noisemakers, the examiner's voice or pure tones.

Gesell and coworkers (3) state that even at a few weeks of age children recognize the mother's voice and experience pleasure on hearing it. A normal child at three months of age tries to turn his head or look at a sound source. Reflex responses to sound are replaced by acquired responses as the child grows older. The child begins to recognize more and more sounds as he grows older and the sounds acquire specific meanings as they are experienced more often. Reflex responses are observed less frequently as the child evidences responses to weaker and weaker sounds. During the latter part of the first year of a child's life, he usually shows definite signs that he can respond consciously to conversational voice and during the second year it becomes possible to utilize auditory tests with spoken sounds, e.g. to urge the child to obey simple instructions. Whispered sounds cannot generally be used until the child has reached two years of age when it should be possible to have the child follow simple whispered requests or to repeat whispered words.

These reactions to auditory stimulation characteristic of different age levels are sometimes used as general guides in the interpretation of responses of infants to gross tests of hearing sensitivity, and in determining whether the child falls within normal limits of response or whether more detailed investigation of his auditory function is necessary.

The presence of the "recruitment" phenomenon may complicate the interpretation of the child's reactions to these gross tests. A youngster with a severe or even a moderate sensorineural hearing loss secondary to cochlear pathology may manifest a marked startle reaction at levels close to his threshold, leading the examiner to conclude that his hearing is normal or close to normal. It should be noted, however, that the presence of recruitment has not been conclusively demonstrated in hypoacusic children.

There is another element of danger in tests involving startle reactions to auditory stimuli. This type of procedure may represent an unpleasant auditory experience for the child, particularly when intense sounds are suddenly and unexpectedly introduced resulting in a reaction of whimpering or crying by the child. It may be difficult for the audiologist and others working with the child to establish rapport for a number of weeks or even months following an initial unpleasant experience in the test situation. Information of limited value regarding the status of the child's hearing may then have been elicited at great cost.

C. Conditioned Reflex Testing Using Pain as Unconditioned Stimulus

Aldrich (4) used sound as one stimulus and pain as the other to establish the hearing status of a three month old baby. At half hour intervals a small dinner bell was rung beside the baby's crib in such a way that she would not see it, while at the same time the sole of the right foot was firmly scratched with a pin. When these stimuli were applied, the child cried out lustily and drew up the right leg. After twelve to fifteen applications, the infant cried and drew up the leg when the bell was rung and the foot was not touched. If the bell was slightly tinkled, the infant's face at once looked worried. The worried look was followed by a cry when the bell was loudly shaken. This test represents the use of a form of conditioned reflex and is similar in some respects to psychogalvanic skin resistance testing which will be discussed later.

UNCALIBRATED SOUND SOURCES

Many physicians, particularly pediatricians and otolaryngologists who are often called upon to determine the status of a child's hearing, utilize a series of *noisemakers* in their office examinations of these youngsters. Noisemakers are also used by some speech and hearing therapists who perform their services in institutions and in private practice where little, if any, calibrated audiological instrumentation is available. Many audiologists in well-equipped audiology centers also employ noisemakers in the early stages of hearing evaluation. These noisemakers include cowbells, snappers, toy telephones, horns, flutes, shakers and whistles which are readily available in toy shops.

There is little objection to exposing the child to these noisemakers in order to observe qualitatively his response to a variety of sounds, to determine whether some degree of residual hearing is present and to prepare the child for more accurate appraisal of his hearing status with auditory stimuli whose intensity and frequency can be controlled. Many of the sounds produced by these noisemakers are of considerable interest to the young child in contrast to pure tones which represent an abstract type of "laboratory" phenomenon unrelated to anything in the child's environment. It is dangerous, however, to draw definitive conclusions about the status of the child's hearing from the use of noisemakers alone, particularly when the intensity and frequency characteristics of the sounds they produce are unknown to the examiner. Some examiners divide their noisemakers into high frequency, mid-frequency and low-frequency sounds purely on the basis of their own subjective reactions to the sounds they produce. An accurate analysis of the frequency spectra of these noisemakers is often very revealing.

A number of studies have reported the inadequacies of typical noisemakers used in hearing evaluation of young children. Clark (5), for example, used a spectrograph to analyze the frequency composition of a series of twenty-four frequently used noisemakers. He recorded "predominant" and "additional" frequencies for each of the toys tested. Of the total number of twenty-four toys tested, fifteen produced frequencies above or below their predominant frequencies and even within the range of predominant frequencies, 5.4 different frequencies were produced that could be considered predominant. In evaluating the frequency count index, ten or more reinforced frequency areas were present in 46.2 per cent of the toys tested. Only five of the toys, or 21 per cent, had fewer than five frequency components. Only one toy, a silver dinner bell, displayed a narrow enough frequency spectrum to be used as an isolated frequency testing device.

The Ewings (6) in England have pioneered in the development of procedures for the evaluation of hearing in the preschool population. They emphasized the use of sounds which are familiar to the child and which are extracted from the daily enviroment. The stimuli employed by them in hearing evaluation of children below two years of age include the "quiet" voice at six feet from the subject, supplemented by such sounds as the tinkle of a teaspoon against the side of a bottle or a cup, light tapping on a door, and soft high-pitched rattles. They have subjected these sounds to intensity and frequency analysis using sound level meters and octave band analyzers. With control of these parameters available to the examiner, the use of noisemakers has value in the quantification of the child's hearing impairment. Even when the results of a frequency and intensity analysis are available, final conclusions on the status of the child's hearing should await the results of calibrated audiometric studies.

One of the present authors (MHM) analyzed the intensity and frequency composition of a series of noisemakers used by the speech and hearing clinicians in a local institution. The results of this analysis are shown in Table I. The output of each toy was recorded at a fixed distance of five inches from the microphone of a General Radio 1551B sound level meter. The "C" or flat scale of the meter was used to determine the overall noise level produced by each of the noisemakers. The sound level meter was connected to a General Radio 1550A octave band analyzer to determine the amount of acoustic energy in the different octave bands. Eight octave bands in the frequency range of 20-10,000 cps were analyzed. The results of the first two bands must be discounted since the ambient noise

TABLE I

Sound Pressure Levels and Frequency Response of Typical Noisemakers

Type of Sound	Sound Level Meter*	20-75 cps	75-150 cps	150-300 cps	300-600 cps	600-1200 cps	1200-2400 cps	2400-4800 cps	4800-10000 cps
Rattleblock	84 db.								
Cowbell	105	70	64	64	78	96	101	100	100
Toy telephone ring	91	56	50	49	54	63	86	86	85
Twirler	102	58	55	64	81	99	96	91	91
Shaker	98	60	53	57	64	94	92	88	80
Horn	94	56	47	48	69	77	78	91	83
Bells	87	68	61	63	65	73	88	94	91
Whistle	98	50	44	46	49	60	97	83	70

* "C" Scale

level of the room in which the tests were made exceeded the amount of acoustic energy produced by the noisemakers.

The analysis performed indicates that all of the noisemakers were extremely complex in their frequency composition. Considerable acoustic energy is present in most of the octave bands studied. Therefore, even if the overall intensity of these noisemakers is controlled by presenting these sounds through a good quality reproducing system with provision for control of the intensity reaching the patient because of the complex frequency spectra of these noisemakers, it is extremely difficult, and for a number of noisemakers impossible, to draw any conclusions as to the frequency characteristics of the loss of hearing present. If the child has normal or near normal hearing in any part of the frequency range in which the noisemakers contain sound energy, he will respond to the stimulus. The information which the use of noisemakers provides is of so general and nonspecific a nature that it can be obtained equally well from the interview and case history taken from the parents.[1] It does not yield the type of definitive, quantitative information on degree and type of hearing loss present which the examiner requires in order to arrive at a meaningful evaluation of the child's communication disorder so that adequate medical, surgical and rehabilitative procedures can be recommended and initiated.

In this chapter a number of gross tests of hearing sensitivity have been considered. It is our opinion that when adequate equipment and personnel are not available in the immediate area where the patient resides, and where parent or physician suspect a hearing problem, that arrangements should be made to have the child evaluated in a center where adequate facilities are available even if this entails expense and inconvenience to the family. The difficulties involved in such a referral are, we feel, justified in order to provide a complete and definitive evaluation of the child's communication disorder. The family physician should encourage the family to sub-

---

[1]A careful case history and interview of the parents should include an attempt to determine how the child responds at home to such sounds as conversational speech at different intensity levels, radio and television, telephone ring, doorbell, toy musical instruments, squeaking doll, etc. The parents are often astute observers of the child's auditory behavior and can provide much useful information for the physician.

mit the child to such a workup and should assist in making a referral to an appropriate facility. He should also request from the agency evaluating the child a detailed report of its findings and recommendations which should then be discussed with the family. Once the local physician is confident that the child has received a comprehensive evaluation by qualified personnel, he should do everything possible to encourage the family to accept the diagnosis which has been made, even when it is a painful and difficult one. Once an adequate evaluation has been performed, the family physician is in a strategic position to discourage the parents from "shopping around" for other opinions and recommendations which may be less difficult to accept.

The "age of specialization" has created a need for an understanding, compassionate but firm counsellor who can interpret the findings from multiple disciplines for the frequently bewildered family. The family physician is in an ideal position to assume this role and should be encouraged to do so. The family physican can help to cushion the shock of a diagnosis of mental retardation or profound hearing loss. He can direct the concern and attention of the parents to the *positive* aspects of the situation, i.e., the child's potential for development in spite of the problem present, and the need for instituting a program of rehabilitation and education suitable for the child. The family physician thus has a two-fold responsibility to both the child and parents. He must first encourage them to secure a comprehensive diagnostic evaluation at a facility having appropriate equipment and staff, and then encourage and assist the parents in accepting the findings and carrying out the recommendations made.

REFERENCES

(1) Hahlbrock, K. H.: Audiometric testing of the acoustic eyelid closure reflex. *Arch. Ohren-Nasen-u. Kehlkopfh., 174*:139, 1959.

(2) Froeschels, E.: Testing hearing of young children. *Arch. Otolaryng., 43*:93, (Feb.) 1946.

(3) Gesell, A., and others: *The First Five Years of Life:* A Guide to the Study of the Preschool Child. Harper, New York, 1940.

(4) Aldrich, C. A.: A new test for hearing in the newborn. *Am. J. Dis. Child., 35*:36, (Jan.) 1928.

(5) Clark, J. P.: Testing the hearing of children with noise makers— a myth. *Except. Child., 22*:326, 1956.

(6) Ewing, A. W. G.: Children with Defective Hearing, in Ellis, M., ed.: *Modern Trends in Diseases of the Ear, Nose and Throat.* Butterworth and Co., Toronto, 1954, chap. V.

Chapter III

PLAY AUDIOMETRY IN HEARING EVALUATION

PLAY AUDIOMETRY is probably the single most valuable means of evaluating the hearing of pre-school children. It consists of making a game of the child's response to various controlled auditory stimuli. Although this approach to hearing evaluation is time-consuming and requires audiologists who are well trained in handling young children, this technique yields the kind of quantitative and qualitative information of the child's hearing status which is most useful in the assessment of the communicative problem present and in planning for appropriate management.

The child is evaluated with this approach in a play situation which is intrinsically pleasant to him. In the process of hearing evaluation by this method much is learned about the child's ability to master new situations and to relate to others. The child is required to cooperate with an adult other than his parents in a relatively structured setting not unlike the situation in which the program of speech and hearing therapy, auditory training and speech reading will be administered should these be required. The communicative problem of the child may well be due in part, or in its entirety, to causes other than hearing loss. During the conditioning sessions the trained examiner is alert for evidence of such factors, particularly those of a psychic or neurologic nature. The time involved in hearing evaluation using conditioning procedures is, in our judgment, a worthwhile expenditure often contributing significantly to the differential diagnosis and helping to prepare the child for the long range program of auditory rehabilitation which may be required.

The most desirable type of sound stimulus, from the point of view of control of frequency and intensity, is a pure tone. Hearing evaluation should also include the use of calibrated speech materials to the greatest extent possible with each child studied. Since the applicability of a variety of therapeutic medical and surgical procedures is dependent upon the type of hearing loss present, both air and bone conduction measurements should be performed whenever a hearing loss is present, to determine whether the loss of hearing is of the conductive or sensorineural type, or whether a combination of both forms is present. If the child's attention span is short, testing should be limited initially to the portion of the frequency range most important in speech development, an effort being made to determine hearing for both air and bone conduction in this range. This information will make it possible to determine the type of loss present and serve as the basis for determining whether medical and/or surgical treatment is appropriate. The frequencies below and above the range important for speech and language development can be tested later.

It has been suggested that some children may not respond to pure tone stimuli because such sounds are unfamiliar and meaningless to them rather than because they are unable to hear them. It has even been suggested that an isolated deafness for pure tones may exist in some children. Froeschels and Beebe (1) investigated the hearing of thirty-three newborn infants aged between half a day and nine days. They used Urbantschitsch's harmonica and tuning forks to determine the motor responses to sound in these newborn infants. They found that although all of the children responded to the harmonica, only one responded to the tuning fork. The Ewings (2) consider the application of pure tone audiometry impossible with children under five years of age because such sounds have little interest to them. We have found that it is possible to make pure tones interesting to the child by comparing them to sounds which are familiar to them. The low frequency sounds can be compared to fog horns and the high frequency sounds to whistles. In a variety of ways, meaning can be imparted to pure tones and children considerably below the age of five can respond satisfactorily to a pure tone test. In addition to pure tones, the examiner uses speech, music, different types of noises and other sounds and compares the child's responses to these sounds with those obtained for pure tones. Such comparative data are useful in ruling out the presence of nonorganic and nonperipheral pathology which may be present. With adolescents and adults, hearing for speech tends to be better than hearing for pure tones in nonorganic hearing losses (psychogenic deafness and malingering). In central language disturbances such as sensory aphasia and in sensorineural hearing impairments accompanied by severe problems in speech discrimination, hearing for pure tones tends to be better than hearing for speech. Such relationships are difficult to establish in the pre-school child because limitations in speech and languages make the performance of calibrated speech audiometric tests difficult or impossible. A number of procedures for the determination of speech reception thresholds and discrimination scores in children have been developed and will be described later in this chapter under "Speech Audiometry in a Play Situation." Such speech audiometric procedures should be performed whenever possible and the results compared with responses to pure tone testing. The availability of both pure tone and speech audiometric data will assist in ruling out the presence of the nonorganic and nonperipheral conditions mentioned.

In play audiometry two examiners should be present during the actual hearing test although only one is necessary during the preliminary conditioning sessions. At the time of the test, one examiner operates the equipment in a control room while the other works with the child and remains with him in the test room. Both examiners observe the child's test responses and behavior carefully throughout the session. For optimum training of audiological personnel, the functions performed by the audiologists during the test should be interchanged so that each examiner receives experience in both phases of the evaluation procedure. The two room testing suite for sound field hearing evaluation is shown in Figures 1 and 2.

The director, supervisor or coordinator of the clinic must select carefully those personnel who are to be assigned to this phase of the program. They should be individuals who have demonstrated skill and ability with this population in the past or who evidence potential skill in this area. As mentioned before, some otherwise excellent audiologists find considerable difficulty in relating to and working with young children. They prefer the relative security

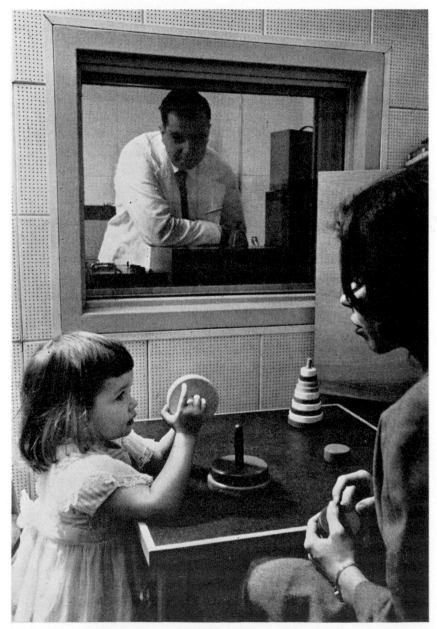

Fig. 1. This figure shows a child being conditioned for a pure tone sound field test. She has been given a block by the audiologist who is teaching her to await the presentation of the pure tone stimulus before placing it on the pole.

(Reproduced with permission of Bernard Cole, Photographer.)

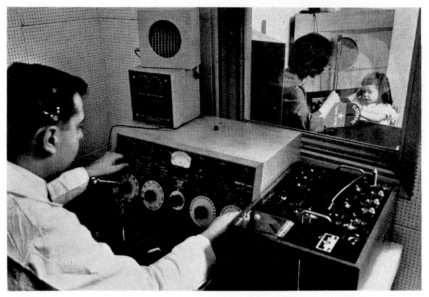

Fig. 2. This figure shows the control room where a second audiologist controls the various stimuli which are presented to the child through one or both loudspeakers in the test room. The monitor microphone in the test room and the loudspeaker in the control room enable the audiologists to communicate with each other during the test. It also permits the audiologist in the control room to hear the child's vocalizations during the examination. (Reproduced with permission of Bernard Cole, Photographer.)

which is possible when testing most adult hard-of-hearing persons from whom specific, quantitative information can be obtained. If a single individual is to render service to all persons with hearing disorders in a given area or institution, the individual who has the responsibility of selecting the audiologist should consider the ability of prospective applicants to work well with young children.

Initial conditioning is performed using pure tones in a sound field thus eliminating the necessity of placing earphones over the child's ears. Many children will accept all phases of the hearing evaluation procedure except the wearing of earphones. These may not be tolerated until greater familiarity with the examiners and the test situation has developed. Some children will accept the wearing of earphones at a very early stage if they are unpretentiously and unceremoniously placed over the ears by a friendly but firm examiner who performs this act in a matter-of-fact manner as a routine part of the evaluation. An occasional child will accept one earphone but not two and the single earphone in this event can be removed from the headband and held against the child's ear by a parent or a member of the staff. The skilled and experienced examiner usually finds little difficulty in determining when and whether earphones can be introduced and will do so at the earliest possible time so that specific information as to the hearing function of each ear can be obtained. It should be remembered that the sound field test is a bilateral test and yields information only about the status of the better-hearing ear.

The important information on the type of hearing loss present which the examiner obtains by a comparison of air and bone conduction thresholds of an impaired ear can be determined only when *earphone* testing is performed for air conduction measurements and a bone conduction vibrator is used to determine the status of the sensorineural portion of the hearing mechanism. Sound field measurements using calibrated sound stimuli are of value in determining whether hearing loss plays a role in the child's communication disorder. They are also useful in establishing the severity and frequency characteristics of the loss present.

When pure tones are introduced into a sound field in the preliminary stages of the hearing evaluation, problems of standing wave patterns are usually encountered. Standing waves from the loudspeaker(s) hit the walls of the test room and are reflected back with the result that some of the sounds will be reinforced and others cancelled. The frequencies which are affected will depend upon the acoustical characteristics of the particular test room. The effects of standing wave patterns can be demonstrated by listening to a continuously presented pure tone in the sound field. As the head is moved from right to left and up and down, some of the tones will appear to change in loudness. This problem is more serious in some testing rooms than in others. It can be satisfactorily resolved by the use of a frequency modulated signal in which the frequency of the sound is periodically altered by controlled amounts usually up 5 per cent of the basic frequency. This feature is available with some of the newer hearing evaluation units and can be added as an accessory to some of the older units. Frequency modulation is an effective way of breaking up standing wave patterns and should be utilized whenever pure tone testing is performed in a sound field.

Any of a variety of types of responses may be accepted in the testing of young children. The response should be *definite* and easily identified as occurring in response to the auditory stimulus. Furthermore, the response should be observable to persons other than the examiner working with the child.

A number of paedo-audiologists employ *indefinite* responses, such as change of expression by the child, cessation of play activity, smiling or laughing, eye movements or pressure of the head against the earphone held by the examiner. The use of such responses should be discouraged and no definitive conclusions about the child's hearing drawn from them. Some of these actions might easily occur spontaneously during the test situation entirely independent of the auditory stimulus, while other responses, such as pressure against the earphone can be experienced only by the examiner working with the child and cannot be confirmed by other persons. The challenging nature of hearing evaluation of young children has encouraged a number of audiologists to specialize in testing this segment of the clinic population, a concentration of professional interest which is encouraged by other audiologists who prefer not to work with a pediatric population. Some of the persons who have specialized in the hearing evaluation of young children have developed great clinical insight which, they feel, makes it possible for them to "know instinctively" when the child does and does not hear a particular sound. Many of these persons rely heavily upon the type of questionable responses previously illustrated. While clinical intuition and insight are qualities "devoutly to be wished," there is danger in accepting hearing evaluations which are based primarily upon subjective reactions and which support rather than test the clinical impressions of the examiner. The uncontrolled use of subjective reactions observable only to a single examiner should be discouraged as vigorously as possible.

Among the test responses which can be utilized in hearing evaluation of children are the following: placing rings on a toy peg, placing cars in a box, dropping blocks in a basket, banging pegs into a board, etc. Such responses can be checked by the examiner operating the test equipment as well as by the audiologist who is with the child so that conclusions on the status of the child's hearing can be jointly determined by two trained observers. The choice among types of responses should not be a rigid one in which the examiner imposes his own preference on the child. Some children prefer one mode of response while others require a different type of response. The examiner can experiment with different types of responses until he discovers the one which has the greatest appeal to the child under evaluation provided the response meets the criteria described. Some children, particularly the more intelligent and active ones have short attention spans and require a change in the type of response in order to maintain their interest. Occasionally, several changes must be made during the course of the evaluation.

Some children cannot be conditioned regardless of the type of response employed or the length of time taken to perform the evaluation. Such children usually present problems, other than, or in addition to, reduced hearing sensitivity, which must be considered by the diagnostic team. The inability of a child to be conditioned after several conditioning sessions conducted by skilled examiners is evidence of the presence of a disorder other than, or in addition to, a peripheral hearing impairment.

Parents of preschool children with communication disorders must be prepared for the time-consuming conditioning procedures which are usually necessary to reach a definite diagnosis. They need to understand and appreciate the reasons for the inability of the examiners to test the child's hearing in a single visit and the need for a total evaluation by trained personnel representing several disciplines. The degree of success achieved in this approach to hearing evaluation is completely dependent upon the cooperation of the child. The child who has been overindulged by well-intentioned but misinformed parents and relatives will not be easy to reach and will need to adjust to the relatively structured setting of the test situation. Unlike many medical examinations which can be performed to some extent without the active cooperation of the child, the audiologist must win the confidence and cooperation of the child before progress in hearing evaluation is achieved.

Some parents find this approach to hearing evaluation difficult to accept. Arrangements for hearing evaluation have been made in many cases upon recommendation of the otolaryngologist following referral of the child by the general practitioner or pediatrician. The parents may have postponed discussion of the suspected hearing loss for many months or years, hoping that their fears and suspicions were unfounded. Other members of the family, frequently the grand-parents, may have assured the parents that all is well and that there is no need to secure professional help. In other cases, the parent may have been bringing the problem to the attention of the family phy-sician for a number of years without his having arranged a referral to an audiology or speech and hearing clinic. Physicians, particularly pediatricians and general practitioners who usually encounter these problems first and who must "live" with the parents who bring these problems to their attention, are too frequently willing to assure the concerned parents that "all is well" and that the child will outgrow the problem. These assurances are usually given without benefit of the results of an adequate evaluation of the child's communication disorder. It is surprising and unfortunate how frequently a physician will fail to consider seriously the parent's complaint that a child's speech does not appear to be normal for his age, or that he fails to respond to auditory stimuli. It is more often the slow speech devel-opment which is ignored, frequently with a casual comment that the child is a "late talker."

Those physicians who are willing to assure the parents that no real problem is present are often men who would never think of dismissing casually a complaint of sore throat, headache or abdominal discomfort without investigating the problem thoroughly. In the area of speech and hearing problems, the family physician often has to be pressed by the parent into arranging for an evaluation. A number of parents, in our experience, have given up trying to con-vince the family physician of the need for an evaluation and have made arrangements on their own for the necessary investigation. Because of the procrastination of the parent or the physician or both, the child is often brought to the speech and hearing clinic months or years after the problem was first noticed. The parent has often delved into the literature on hearing and speech disorders and is superficially cognizant of such terms as "aphasia," "central deafness" and "perceptive hearing loss" and their possible relation to delayed speech in children. The parents are anxious to know "what is wrong" with the child as soon as possible and are hopeful that some form of medical or surgical treatment will rectify the problem. They want specific information and they want it as quickly as possible.

The audiologist's recommendation that a series of visits will be necessary in order to complete the hearing evaluation is often met with disappointment and occasionally with the request that one of the newer techniques of hearing assessment like the "shock test" be used in order to arrive at a diagnosis in the shortest possible time. Most parents will require considerable counselling by trained, understanding personnel at this stage in order to develop an appreciation of: (a) the multiple factors which can contribute to communication disorders in children, each of which must be carefully and systematically explored by trained specialists using appropriate testing techniques, and (b) the desirability of evaluating the child's hearing in as pleasant and non-traumatic a situation as possible, usually over a period of at least several visits. The first of these objectives must be accomplished without unduly alarming the parent or suggesting possible contributory factors which may not exist in the case of a particular child. The complexity of the diagnostic problem must be patiently and diplomatically presented to the parent. The need to "rule out" certain factors which can contribute to communication disorders is presented to the parent in an effort to enlist maximum cooperation without causing undue alarm.

The audiologist may encourage the cooperation of the parent(s) in training the child to respond consistently to auditory stimuli. A cooperative, intelligent, reasonably well-adjusted parent can render considerable assistance by working with the child at home, using the type of response which can then be employed by the audiologists in the test situation. Such supplementary home practice and conditioning techniques may shorten the number of clinic visits required. However, the audiologist must "select" his parents with great care for such home training. Certain parents are too emotionally involved in the child's problem and are too anxious and tense to provide the relaxed home atmosphere which is necessary for supplementary home training. Some parents are riddled by a sense of guilt, invariably unjustified, that they are the cause of the child's speech and hearing problem, or that damage may have resulted from excessive delay in investigating the problem. Such parents may easily do more harm than good in the evaluation program and should be relegated to a supportive rather than an active role in the process. The paedo-audiologist must be able to work with people as well as with instruments. He must be capable of evaluating the emotional adjustment of the parents as well as the communication disorder of the child. On the basis of careful interview with the parents, a decision will be reached as to whether the services of a particular parent should or should not be utilized in conditioning training in the home.

Many children with communication disorders are "dragged" from one specialist to another and from one institution to another. Too often we seem intent on pressing our own prized diagnostic labels on these children to the exclusion of the labels of our colleagues rather than emphasizing to the parents that which is common to our impressions and recommendations. Diagnostic squabbles are often very effectively resolved by astute observation over a period of time of the child's development and response to multiple rehabilitive procedures.

A number of specialists in hearing evaluation of young children have developed various modifications in the clinical application of conditioning procedures. Members of the staff of the John Tracy Clinic in California have developed procedures for hearing evaluation of children under five years of age which have yielded a high degree of clinical accuracy as verified by longitudinal studies of children with different degrees of hearing loss. (3) The child initially learns to make a response to a drum beat which he can see and also feel. The drum beat is later sounded without the child seeing the drum. After the response is learned, the tones from a standard pure tone audiometer are substituted for the drum. The testing is performed in a play situation with a series of toys which are changed frequently enough to maintain the child's attention. These play activities include such responses as placing rings on a peg, cars in a box, and the like. The method of response to the auditory stimulus is first demonstrated to the child by the examiner. The examiner shows approval when the child makes a correct response to the sound presented. The procedures employed in hearing evaluation of pre-schoolers at the John Tracy Clinic are presented in a twenty minute film entitled "Too Young To Say." The authors have found this film valuable for a variety of teaching purposes including presentations to audiologists, speech therapists, nurses, medical students, physicians and parents.

Barr (4) tested almost 300 children ranging in age from one to six years using psychogalvanic skin resistance combined with play audiometry. A single examiner is used in the play audiometry situation described by Barr. The child sits at a small table beside the audiometer, obliquely across from the operator who observes the child constantly. The operator controls the tone interrupter with the right hand and gives the child play instructions with the left. The right hand is hidden behind a screen constructed so as to prevent the child from learning by seeing the movements of the operator's hand that a tone has been presented. The tones are usually presented directly to the child's ear via an earphone but, in isolated cases, teaching has been started with the tones presented from a loud-speaker when the child rejects the earphone. Barr emphasizes the confidence which the child must have in the examiner.

Auditory measurement must not be started until complete confidence and trust have been established between the child and the tester. On the table, in front of the child, a simple colorful toy is placed. These are of the educational toy type, such as a nest of round or square boxes that fit one inside the other, or a game of the Chinese checkers type in which the holes in a game board are filled with marbles. The child can select from a box a group of small animals that can be collected into a menagerie or farm yard. The toys in their combination possibilities must be adapted to the greatest extent possible to the developmental level and personal taste of the individual child. The most important factor is that these toys can be used for what may be called a "series" game.

Barr suggests that conditioning be started by giving the child a tone at an intensity level which, from previous observation, he may be expected to hear. When the tone is presented, the operator simultaneously indicates with a quick, sharp, definite motion that, for example, a marble should be taken from the box and placed in a hole on the Chinese checker board. The operator's simple, concise instructions should be given in a demonstrative manner if the child is to understand the meaning of the game. The instructions are repeated as many times as necessary and the child is encouraged to "help" move the marble. Gradually, the child is allowed to carry out the entire little demonstration himself. If he tries to move a marble when no tone has been sounded, he is *immediately* stopped. The moving of the marble thus becomes a kind of reward for the perception of and response to the tone. It is important that the "games" be changed from time to time to retain the child's interest. The whole procedure must be kept interesting if the best results are to be obtained. When it is certain that the child has learned the object of the game, the threshold determination is starte^r, i.e., the tone intensity is varied in the usual manner. When all frequencies of importance to the diagnosis have been tested with one ear the opposite ear is then examined.

SPECIAL PURE TONE CONDITIONING TECHNIQUES

Several specialized test procedures have been developed to elicit and retain the interest and cooperation of a young child during the hearing evaluation. Some of these are described in the following pages.

A.   The Peep Show

One of the best known of these procedures is the Peep Show (5, 6) developed by Dix and Hallpike in England. This technique has received enthusiastic acceptance by workers in a number of institutions and is worthy of the serious attention and consideration of all persons concerned with hearing evaluation in young children. The originators of this procedure believe that a child should have reached a mental age of three years in order for this technique to be applicable to him.

Dix and Hallpike were concerned with the development of a test procedure which would insure an accurate measure of hearing capacity in children in the course of a single visit. The Peep Show apparatus is divided into two parts and is illustrated in Figure 3. Part

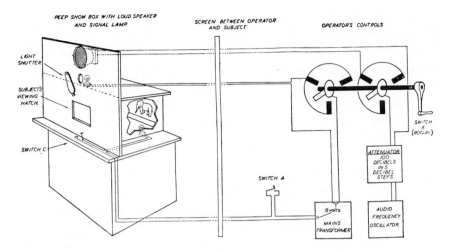

Fig. 3. Diagram of the Peep Show test apparatus.

1 of the instrumentation is operated by the child and consists of a wooden box with a picture at the rear which is well suited to the age and interests of the child being tested. This picture can be seen through a viewing hatch when illuminated by means of an electric light bulb. Above the viewing hatch is another bulb, which can be seen through a shuttered orifice and above this orifice is a loudspeaker. The bulb is a signal lamp, and is used with the loudspeaker to give a synchronized visual and auditory signal. It thus serves to facilitate conditioning as does the associated visual and auditory presentation of the drum in the conditioning procedures used at the John Tracy Clinic. As soon as possible during the Peep Show test, the visual cue is removed and the auditory stimulus alone is presented. The use of a combined visual and auditory stimulus is based upon procedures developed by experimental psychologists and facilitates the conditioning process. This portion of the Peep Show apparatus is used and operated by the child who is seated in front of the viewing hatch.

The child is separated by a screen from part 2 of the apparatus which is used by the tester. The screen has a hole in it through which the tester can view the subject without himself being observed. The tester's armamentarium is composed of a pure tone generator and an attenuator together with a transformer whose output is eight volts. The output leads of the tone generator and transformer pass to the double rotary switch B which is operated by a single handle. From the switch, the two pairs of leads pass respectively to the loudspeaker and signal lamp of the subject's apparatus. These provide a synchronized visual and auditory signal when the handle of switch B is rotated by the tester. An additional eight volt tapping from the transformer supplies the illumination bulb in the picture box. The leads reach it by way of two press-button switches arranged in series. One of these, switch A, is controlled by the tester. The other, switch C is controlled by the child. The picture is illuminated only when the two switches are pressed simultaneously. The child is thus rewarded by the sight of the picture when he presses the switch in association with the presentation of the sound stimulus.

The details of the instrumentation used by the designers of the Peep Show are included here because the instrument is not commercially available at the present time. Readers desirous of utilizing this approach to hearing evaluation must therefore make their own arrangements for building the necessary equipment. The electrical components and other materials required are inexpensive and readily available. This equipment can be prepared by the clinician with a knowledge of simple electronics or by a technician whose services are usually available in hospitals and medical centers.

The test procedure suggested by Dix and Hallpike is as follows: after the child's cooperation has been elicited, he is seated with his face two feet from the viewing hatch. Switch C is within easy reach of his right hand. An examiner sits at the child's left and focuses the child's attention on the signal lamp. The examiner observes and notes when the child's attention is on the lamp. He then rotates switch B and presses switch A thereby producing simultaneous impulses from the lamp and the loudspeaker. A 1000 cps tone is used at a level of 80 db. re normal threshold. When the two signals go on, the examiner presses switch C which lights up the picture. The examiner then stops the rotation of switch B, opens switch A and the picture, light and sound disappear. The instructor takes his hand off switch C.

This process is then repeated until the child has learned to press switch C by himself. The lamp signal is then withdrawn and the tone alone is presented. The tester repeats the signal presentation reducing the intensity by 20 db. with each successive presentation until there is no response. The intensity is then raised in 10 db. steps until a response reappears. The threshold is then recorded on a standard audiogram form. Calibration is determined by using a normal hearing person whose head is placed in the same position as that of the child. Since the presentation of pure tones through a loudspeaker presents a number of acoustic problems which may interfere with the validity of the test including the problem of standing wave patterns, it is desirable to use a frequency-modulated tone when the auditory stimulus is presented. The same procedure is used to determine threshold at the other test frequencies. The child is reconditioned with both the signal light and the sound at each new frequency.

The authors claim that the entire testing procedure generally lasts from ten to fifteen minutes. Children show no signs of fatigue or boredom providing the pictures are changed. Thresholds can be repeated with regularity and the tester requires no great skill. Dix and Hallpike believe their test procedure requires that the child have at least normal intelligence and be at least three years of age. The procedure is especially well suited for intelligent, active youngsters who are frequently bored by standard pure tone audiometry and whose interest may wane after several minutes of testing. The Peep Show approach to hearing evaluation permits the examiner to change the picture used in the viewing hatch and thus maintain the interest of the child under test.

A number of useful modifications of the above procedure have been developed. Denmark (7) describes the Peep Show which he designed for use at the Liverpool School for the Deaf in Lancashire. Instead of the hand rotated drum of Dix and Hallpike, a silent motor driven turntable rotates a roundabout which is brightly colored. A moving object is much more interesting to a child than a still picture and is incorporated into the Denmark modification. The entire instrument is in a box which can be placed on any table and connected to any pure tone audiometer without special modifications of the circuit of the instrument. Each ear is tested separately with earphones in the Denmark modification thus providing more valuable diagnostic information than a bilateral sound field test. A small screen hides the tester's hands and a silent switch requiring only a light touch is provided. The procedure as described by Denmark requires only one examiner rather than two as described by Dix and Hallpike. Denmark uses the Peep Show when he is unable to obtain what he considers consistent results with conventional pure tone audiometry. The Peep Show, according to Denmark, requires no preliminary explanation and attracts and maintains the child's attention so that he responds more positively to small auditory sensations near threshold and more accurate results are therefore obtained.

Shimizu and Nakamura (8) have introduced a lantern slide test in which pictures are thrown on a screen in a sound proof room if the child presses a button when he hears a tone. This represents still another modification of the original Peep Show test of Dix and Hallpike. In the Shimizu-Nakama version, the visual portion of the test is adapted to the interests of the modern, electronically oriented child who tends to become disinterested in still pictures. The original Peep Show requires a fixed posture as the child observes a hole in a box. The lantern slide test, on the other hand, permits the child greater freedom of movement. This is a real advantage for the hyperactive child and for those with short attention spans. In a group of ten children with known normal hearing, Shimizu and Nakama found a difference of 10-15 db. between the "exact" threshold and that determined by the lantern slide test. They do not consider this to be a significant deviation since young children generally do not respond to test tones at threshold levels. They have found the test most successful as have Dix and Hallpike with children over three years of age and report no success with the very young child.

Statten and Wishart (9) consider the Peep Show an extremely valuable technique for hearing evaluation in children. Their Peep Show apparatus is in the form of an attractively colored doll's house which contains a standard pure tone audiometer with earphones. A loudspeaker is mounted on the doll's house. A movie projector is incorporated in the assembly which throws an image on a ground glass screen situated down the hallway, inside the open front door. Over the doorway is a porch light and beside it is a doorbell. When the tones are sounded, pressing the doorbell will start the motion picture. The porch light serves as the visual signal to aid conditioning. The motion picture used is in color and was taken on a farm showing familiar animals and scenes.

The Statten-Wishart Peep Show assembly is far more exciting to the child than the simpler assembly used by Dix and Hallpike. Instead of an unexciting light bulb, Statten and Wishart have transformed the visual signal into a meaningful porch light. The film they show is of greater interest to youngsters reared in rural areas than to city children to whom farm life may be very unfamiliar. For the urban child, a motion picture showing skyscrapers, subways and construction equipment might be of more interest, or would at least be more familiar. Statten and Wishart felt that some children might be frightened by the activity of a movie and so provided a slide projector to show colored still pictures for such children. Experience has shown that the motion pictures are preferred by a majority of the children.

An ideal approach to the use of the Peep Show procedure involves a combination of the motion picture technique suggested by Statten and Wishart with the approach suggested by Shimizu and Nakama. In the combined approach, the child presses a button and starts a movie which is projected on a screen. The excitement and interest of a motion picture would be combined with the freedom of movement desirable and necessary for testing some children. Both earphones and a loudspeaker should be available to the examiner. The loudspeaker is used for children unable to tolerate earphones at the time of initial testing. We feel that the services of two examiners is desirable for this test as suggested by Dix and Hallpike in order to provide greater control of the test situation and to reduce the subjective interpretation of questionable responses which often occurs when one examiner performs all of the functions necessary in this type of test.

Green (10) describes the "Pup Show" which is another adaptation of the Peep Show in which the motivational device used is a toy dog. To begin the test, the child's fingers are placed near but not touching the button switch which is wired to the toy dog. When the child is ready, a tone calculated to be well above threshold is presented and the child is helped to manipulate the button in order to activate the dog. This is repeated several times until the child has become conditioned to give this response. After conditioning has occurred, the tester proceeds with both air and bone conduction tests as in conventional audiometry. All of the necessary parts of the apparatus with the exception of the audiometer can be purchased quite inexpensively. The apparatus which is attached to the audiometer is compact and portable and may be unplugged and stored when not in use.

Sullivan, Miller and Polisar (11) have reported still another simplified version of the Peep Show in which the entire cost of the apparatus is less than four dollars. The main feature of this version of the test is that the push button apparatus of the pure tone audiometer is used by the child under test to activate a toy dog similar to that used by Green. The patient signal device is an accessory of many commercially available pure tone audiometers but is frequently not utilized by many testers who prefer a hand-raising response. No special changes or modifications of the circuit of the audiometer are required. While we do not find this test approach necessary for most children, it has proven of value in evaluating the hearing of active, intelligent youngsters whose attention it is difficult to maintain with conventional procedures. It is particularly applicable to children between the ages of 3 and 5 years. The portable Pup Show is shown in use in Figure 4.

B.   Pediacoumeter (Puppet Show Hearing Test)

Guilford and Haug (12) developed an instrument known as the Pediacoumeter for testing the hearing of children two to six years of age. The instrument is an electrically-powered, solenoid-operated portable device which is used in conjunction with a conventional pure tone audiometer. Seven jack-in-the-box heads have been appropriately modified to represent each of the audiometric test tones and attached to the solenoids for release by the push button switch in the hands of the child tested. In addition, a solenoid switch is provided for the tester.

Two types of test procedures are used with the Pediacoumeter. The first is the "normal" test which is used for children over three

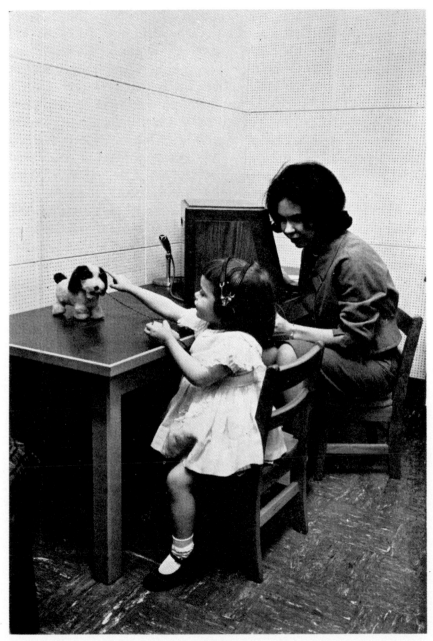

Fig. 4. The modified Pup Show in clinical use. (Reproduced with permission of Bernard Cole, Photographer.)

years of age where there is no indication of "total" hearing loss, or of mental or emotional disturbance. The child is told that he will play a game with little houses and people in them. He is to press the button when he hears the "little person" asking to get out. A red light flashes if the child presses the button when the tone is not being presented so that he can be discouraged from random playing. We have found that the red light does not fulfill this purpose but acts instead as a type of visual reward which appeals to some children as much as the true reward. The removal of the visual signal following random pressing of the button in the Peep Show is, in our experience, a more desirable arrangement. When the child hears the sound he presses the button and out pops a head. The examiner works with 5 db. decrements in the intensity of the tones until thresholds are determined at each of the test frequencies.

The second version of this test is a "conditioning" approach and is used when the chronological age is below three years and when there is a possibility of total deafness or insufficient auditory or perceptual maturity. The objective of testing these children is not to obtain a complete audiogram but to determine whether they can hear and to ascertain the general degree of impairment which is present. In this form of Pediacoumeter test, the tone is presented well above threshold with the tester switch closed. After repeated presentations, the child recognizes that the sound stimulus and the light, plus pressing his button, result in the popping up of the jack-in-the-box. The light is removed, and if the push button response remains when the sound is presented, it is assumed that the child has heard the test tone. The reverse assumption, however, is not valid since the child may hear the sound but not respond because of the presence of other, nonauditory disturbances, such as mental retardation or neurological disorder.

Guilford and Haug find the test practical, easy to administer and a reliable clinical tool for testing children because of its interest appeal. They record a threshold variation of 0-10 db. for the Pediacoumeter compared to a variation of 0-50 db. for conventional audiometry. They report an average difference range on retest for any given frequency of 2.1-4.2 db. compared to a range of 19.2-34.3 db. for standard pure tone testing. In their hands, therefore, the

Pediacoumeter yields significantly greater reliability than does standard pure tone audiometry for the age group noted.

Waldrop (13) has reported that complete audiograms can be obtained on children between the ages of three to six with this technique. Other workers in the field have encountered differing degrees of success with this approach.

In general, it can be stated that few audiologists are able to equal the success, with a particular mode of testing achieved by the originators of any particular method. The innovators of a test procedure have a degree of enthusiasm, interest and experience with the procedure which cannot be readily equalled by others. Furthermore, these innovators bring to the test situation their unique personal gifts in handling children which cannot entirely be separated from the effectiveness of the method per se. Finally, it should be noted that the initial introduction of a procedure is usually followed by a wave of enthusiasm which is tempered by the clinical experience which follows. Such experience makes it possible to evaluate the technique with the necessary perspective and to weigh objectively its value to the clinician.

For children five years of age or younger, we use play conditioning procedures similar to those employed by the John Tracy Clinic. Testing is performed in a two room testing suite with two examiners present during the evaluation. A variety of sound stimuli including pure tones are presented through a loudspeaker and the child is trained to give a specific response using a variety of serial games. This approach is used *only* when the child is unable to tolerate earphones. Many children below the age of five can respond satisfactorily to a standard pure tone test administered through earphones, and there is no need for sound field testing for them. We have successfully tested many children down to the age of three with this method. In those cases in which sound field testing is necessary, earphones are introduced at the earliest possible time so that information on the status of each ear can be obtained. We then move to bone conduction measurements as soon as possible.

The specialized play conditioning procedures such as the Peep Show and its modifications and the Pediacoumeter have value for some children but we do not find it necessary to use such procedures routinely. The interest of an occasional child can be maintained with one of these specialized approaches but in general we have little difficulty in maintaining his interest with one or more serial games. We do not consider any of these special play audiometric procedures an essential part of the clinical armamentarium. The severely involved child with multiple etiological factors contributing to his communication disorder will frequently be found untestable by either standard or specialized techniques of play audiometry. Of those children who are potentially testable, the most important factors in successful testing are the skill and ingenuity of the examiners, rather than the number or complexity of the test equipment available. Skilled and understanding personnel can do more to retain the interest of the child than any piece of inanimate test apparatus. With this demanding population, at least, no instrument or combination of instruments, regardless of how clever their construction, can replace the skilled and experienced pediatric audiologist.

SPEECH AUDIOMETRY IN A PLAY SITUATION

A number of attempts have been made to apply the techniques of calibrated speech audiometry to children. The major efforts have been directed at determining a hearing threshold for speech (SRT) using test materials appropriate to the age and interests of the child. Recently, efforts have also been made to develop discrimination tests for children.

Keaster (14) described a technique for determining the speech thresholds of children three to six years of age. Twenty five nouns were selected from the first thousand words on the International Kindergarten Word List which is believed to comprise the spoken vocabulary of most children under six years of age. Pictures were then selected to represent the nouns. The examiner reads a list of sentences containing the test words through a calibrated amplifying system whose output is fed through a loudspeaker in the room where the child is seated. The material is initially presented at a level well above the child's probable threshold. The intensity is then reduced until the child is no longer able to respond to the material presented. The lowest level at which the child is able to respond to at least three test stimuli is considered his speech threshold. Several typical items are the following: "Put the *rabbit* on the floor." "Point to the *boat*." "Show the *bird* to the lady." The thresholds obtained by this procedure are not necessarily analagous to the well known speech reception threshold (SRT) obtained with adults.

Siegenthaler and associates (15) describe a similar picture identification test for determining speech thresholds in children. Monosyllabic nouns are used with accompanying pictures. The items selected are familiar to children three and four years of age, phonetically dissimilar, representative of speech sounds, and homogeneous in basic audibility. The authors claim that the results of their test correlate well with the average pure tone hearing loss for a group of children.

There is considerable danger in substituting a speech threshold test for a pure tone test for the purpose of detecting and measuring hearing loss in children, or, for that matter, in adults. While the pure tone stimulus is discrete as to frequency, speech is a complex signal containing many frequencies which change rapidly as a function of time. Spondee words have their critical acoustic energy below 1000 cps. Persons with normal hearing up to 1000 cps and a marked high frequency loss have little difficulty in a test of spondee words or one which employs numbers. Significant high frequency losses of hearing thus escape detection when speech material is used in which the vowels are the key phonetic elements. This has proved to be a major limiting factor in the whispered and spoken voice tests and in the "fading numbers" test. (16) Specially prepared material for use in determining the speech thresholds of children are, however, of value when performed *in addition to* pure tone audiometry.

Myatt and Landes (17) reported a picture identification test to determine the discrimination ability of children. The key words were selected from the Thorndike lists which contain material familiar to children. The words were analyzed and grouped according to phonetic composition similar to the manner in which the standard PB-50 lists are used for testing discrimination ability in adults. Landes believes that his test represents the first attempt to apply the picture-identification technique to the determination of discrimination ability.

Three lists of kindergarten phonetically balanced word lists have been prepared by Haskins (18) and contain simple, familiar words suitable for testing children. They can be used in place of the standardized adult lists which are the Psycho-Acoustic Laboratory PB-50 and the Central Institute for the Deaf W-22 Lists. Among the words included on the kindergarten PB lists (PBK's) are "please," "cage," "peg" and "camp." The value of discrimination testing has been well documented and comprises a routine part of the audiological evaluation of adult hard of hearing patients. It should similarly be part of the audiological evaluation of children whenever such testing is possible.

REFERENCES

(1) Froeschels, E. and Beebe, H.: Testing the hearing of new born infants. *Arch. Otolaryng., 44*:710, (Dec.) 1946.

(2) Ewing, I. R., and Ewing, A. W. G.: The ascertainment of deafness in infancy and early childhood. *J. Laryng. and Otol., 59*:309, (Sept.) 1944.

(3) Lowell, E., Rushford, G., Hoverston, G. and Stoner, M.: Evaluation of pure tone audiometry with preschool age children. *J. Speech and Hearing Disorders, 21*:292, (Sept.) 1956.

(4) Barr, B.: Pure tone audiometry for pre-school children; a preliminary report. *Acta Otolaryng.*, Supp. *110*:89, 1954.

(5) Dix, M. R. and Hallpike, C. S.: Peep-Show; new technique for pure-tone audiometry in young children. *Brit. M. J., 2*:719, (Nov. 8) 1947.

(6) Dix, M. R. and Hallpike, C. S.: Peep-Show audiometry. *Proceedings of the Third World Congress of the Deaf*, Wiesbaden, 1959, p. 127.

(7) Denmark, F. G. W.: A development of the peep-show audiometer. *J. Laryng. and Otol., 64*:357, 1950.

(8) Shimizu, H. and Nakamura, F.: Pure-tone audiometry in children; lantern-slides test. *Ann. Otol. Rhin. and Laryng., 66*:392, (June) 1957.

(9) Statten, P. and Wishart, D. E. S.: Pure-tone audiometry in young children; psychogalvanic-skin-resistance and peep show. *Ann. Otol. Rhin. and Laryng., 65*:511, (June) 1956.

(10) Green, D. S.: The pup show: a simple inexpensive modification of the peep show. *J. Speech and Hearing Disorders, 23*:118 (Feb.) 1958.

(11) Sullivan, R., Miller, M. H. and Polisar, I. A.: The portable pup-show: a further modification of the pup-show. *Arch. Otolaryng., 76*:49, (July) 1962.

(12) Guilford, F. R. and Haug, C. O.: Diagnosis of deafness in the very young child. *A.M.A. Arch. Otolaryng., 55*:101 (Feb.) 1952.

(13) Waldrop, W. F.: Puppet show hearing test. *Volta Review, 55*:488, (Dec.) 1953.

(14) Keaster, J.: A quantitative method of testing the hearing of young children. *J. Speech Disorders, 12*:159, (June) 1947.

(15) Siegenthaler, B. M., Pearson, J. and Lezak, R. J.: A speech reception threshold test for children. *J. Speech and Hearing Disorders, 19*:360, (Sept.) 1954.

(16) Fowler, E. P., Jr.: Discovery and evaluation of otic cripples. *Arch. Otolaryng., 45*:550, (May) 1947.

(17) Myatt, B. D. and Landes, B. A.: Assessing discrimination loss in children; a new approach toward a picture test. *Arch. Otolaryng., 77*:359, (Apr.) 1963.

(18) Haskins, H. L.: Kindergarten PB word lists in Newby, H. A.: *Audiology: Principles and Practice.* Appleton-Century-Crofts, New York, 1958, p. 327.

Chapter IV

ELECTROPHYSIOLOGICAL AUDIOMETRY

Special auditory tests have been developed to evaluate the hearing of young children who cannot be tested with the conventional procedures previously described. The procedures which we have considered thus far require, for the most part, the active cooperation of the child under test. They involve play-conditioning and require that the child be "conditionable." The child must be able and willing to give a voluntary response to the auditory stimuli. Modifications of basic play-audiometric procedures such as the Peep Show and the Pediacoumeter require that the child have at least normal intelligence. Children with communication disorders secondary to conditions other than, or in addition to, reduced hearing sensitivity are extremely difficult and, in some cases impossible, to evaluate audiologically by standard subjective procedures.

The electrophysiological procedures which have been developed to evaluate hearing in children are highly specialized and should be performed only in audiology centers functioning as part of a medical institution where the services of all the essential professional personnel are available. We do not consider these procedures "routine" and they do not constitute part of the basic examination battery performed on children with communication disorders. They are, instead, highly specialized methods which should be used with discretion for certain children. When these procedures are utilized, they are always part of a total evaluation and should never be performed separate from other forms of investigation.

The two types of electrophysiological procedures which have been developed for the purpose of evaluating hearing in children are psychogalvanic skin resistance testing and electroencephalographic testing. A discussion of these techniques follows.

[50]

PSYCHOGALVANIC SKIN RESISTANCE TESTING (PGSR)
or
ELECTRODERMAL AUDIOMETRY (EDA)

Recently the term "electrodermal audiometry" (EDA) (1) has been suggested as being more appropriate than the better known psychogalvanic skin resistance audiometry (PGSR). In this text we will employ the older, more familiar designation, PGSR.

Psychogalvanic skin resistance testing is based upon the Feré effect and Pavlovian conditioned responses. The Feré effect has been known since 1888 and refers to a change in the electrical resistance between two points on the surface of the skin. This can be measured and recorded, and is part of the basis of PGSR testing (2). This change in skin resistance occurs, however, only in response to intense sounds and is thus of limited value in the determination of auditory thresholds. To be clinically useful a response is required which can be evoked by near-threshold sounds. Pavlovian conditioning makes it possible to utilize changes in skin resistance to obtain near-threshold responses.

When the sympathetic nervous system is stimulated, an increase in the activity of the sudoriferous (sweat) glands occurs. A mild faradic shock is used to stimulate the sympathetic nervous system. It will be recalled that Pavlov's early experiments involved the use of dogs in whom salivation (unconditioned response) occurred in association with the presentation of food (unconditioned stimulus). A bell (conditioned stimulus) was sounded before the presentation of the food. After several trials the dogs salivated when the bell was sounded, in anticipation of the food. In PGSR audiometry, sweating is the unconditioned response which follows the presentation of the faradic shock (unconditioned stimulus). The conditioned stimulus is a pure tone. After several tone-shock presentations, sweating occurs following the presentation of the tone alone in anticipation of the shock. When this occurs, conditioning has been achieved and a complete pure tone audiogram can be obtained according to standard clinical procedures. Hardy, Pauls and Bordley of the Hearing and Speech Center of Johns Hopkins Medical Center are responsible for applying the phenomena of skin resistance changes to the testing of hearing in young children and for evolving a practical clinical procedure. These authors have contributed a series of highly important papers to the literature describing different aspects of PGSR testing in children. (3, 4) Their important work in this area serves as the basis for the use of this approach to hearing evaluation in children which is now employed in many audiology centers throughout the world.

The basic instrumentation for the performance of this test described by Hardy and his associates at Johns Hopkins is that developed by Richter in the Phipps Psychobiologic Laboratory. (5, 6, 7, 8) In these references will be found a description of the apparatus and procedure which Hardy and associates applied to the testing of hearing in young children. Richter was able to demonstrate skin resistance changes with his equipment in a variety of normal and pathologic states following such external stimuli as pin pricks, strong light and mild faradic shock. Hardy experimented with a variety of stimuli and found that a mild faradic shock produced the most consistent conditioning.

The idea of PGSR testing as described by Hardy is that, with the use of a pure tone as a warning signal a few seconds before a shock is administered, a child can be conditioned so that significant skin resistance changes are developed following the presentation of the tone in anticipation of the shock. Hardy implies that the sweating response is analagous to the finger raising response in adults. "Instead of raising a finger or moving a toy, the child sweats if the tone is heard." The conclusion which can be reached from this statement is that the results of PGSR audiometry are interchangeable with those of subjective testing. This conclusion is questioned by Bordley (9) and others who consider PGSR testing as a measure of sub-cortical hearing and not equivalent to behavioral responses. Behavioral audiometry in contrast to PGSR measurement involves the conscious, volitional participation of the subject. Bordley believes that the auditory-sympathetic reflex lies below the cortex and above the level of the inferior colliculi and the rostral border of the pons. A PGSR audiogram therefore would represent a test of the efficiency of the auditory pathway up to that point, rather than a measure of the integrity of the entire auditory mechanism.

The localization of the region in the brain for the mediation of the galvanic skin reflex to auditory stimuli has not been established. Bordley (10) emphasizes the importance of determining the lowest level of communication between the auditory pathways and the sympathetic nervous system. In 1954, Wang, working in Richter's laboratory, established the level of the shock-sweat reflex in cats by transection of the brain at the intercollicular level to the rostral border of the pons. Transection above this level did not abolish the reflex. Bordley concludes that the auditory-sympathetic reflex must lie somewhere below the cortex and above the level of the inferior colliculi and the rostral border of the pons.

These findings are based upon animal research and may not be directly applicable to PGSR measurements in man. The localization of the auditory-galvanic reflex in the human has not been definitely established. It is possible that the cerebral cortex plays a more important role in this reflex in man than in animals and that an intact cortex is necessary for PGSR responses. Comparative physiology suggests increased "encephalization" as we move to higher evolutionary levels with man representing a greater concentration of function at the cortical level than in any of the lower species. It is therefore difficult to extrapolate data from animal research in this area to the human level. It is, of course, also possible that while the reflex pathway may be at the same level in man, his higher centers being better developed might well modify (as the cat might not) this shock-sweat response.

A number of clinical studies suggest that the results of PGSR and subjective audiometry are *not* interchangeable. Bordley and Haskins (10, 11) reported a series of audiological characteristics of presbyacusic patients with nonperipheral pathology. One of the audiological characteristics of such patients is better hearing as measured by PGSR audiometry than by subjective or behavioral tests. A number of workers are testing children with *both* PGSR and subjective methods. The implication of this dual approach is that the disparity between results of these two modes of evaluation is a quantitative measure of the degree of nonperipheral hearing impairment which is present. The Portmanns, (12) for example, consider PGSR audiometry, in spite of its limitations, a practical clinical procedure. They interpret recent work on the conditioned reflex as an indication that only lesions of the cochlea, the eighth nerve, the acoustic centers, and the mesencephalon will be reflected in losses on a PGSR audiogram. Results of psychogalvanometry, they believe, should be interpreted with extreme caution whenever one deals with deafness of central origin.

PGSR audiometry may prove to be of greatest value by providing information about the status of the peripheral hearing mechanism. That the results are not infrequently at variance with those of subjective methods should not be considered a weakness of this test modality.

PGSR testing requires consummate skill and experience on the part of the examiners. It has fallen into some disrepute because it has been employed by individuals with inadequate understanding of the technique who were unable to interpret the results as a part of the total evaluation of the child. The publicity given this technique in lay publications and other mass media has resulted in a demand on the part of some parents that their child be administered the "shock test" even when it is possible to evaluate the child's hearing satisfactorily by conventional techniques. Other parents have developed unreasoned fears about the test believing that it will result in physical or psychological harm to the child. These fears can be easily allayed in most cases by a simple explanation to the parents of the essentials of the test and of the contribution it can make to the accurate diagnosis of the child's problem.

PGSR audiometry is not the panacea which some workers expected it to be on the basis of the initially overoptimistic reports which appeared in the literature. The procedure, unfortunately, proves to be of least value in those cases where it is most necessary. Children who are difficult to condition by standard play audiometric techniques usually turn out to be difficult to test by PGSR audiometry. Initial expectations from PGSR testing have given way to a more realistic appraisal of the clinical value of this technique.

An important application of PGSR audiometry is in the evaluation of adults with suspected nonorganic or functional hearing losses, i.e., malingering and psychogenic deafness. Audiology centers operated by the United States Armed Forces and the Veterans Administration make extensive use of PGSR audiometry where the problem of detection of nonorganic hearing impairment is a major one. The technique is also of value in medico-legal cases where, for example, hearing loss is claimed as a result of an industrial accident or exposure to high intensity noise. In the Veterans Administration audiology centers PGSR testing is routinely performed at one or more frequencies. (1)

The application of PGSR audiometry to the evaluation of hearing in young children is fraught with important clinical and theoretical problems, a number of them as yet unresolved. That PGSR tests the integrity of the peripheral pathway in contrast to standard subjective audiometry has already been mentioned. A number of practical clinical problems also exist in PGSR audiometry. Extraneous physical movements must be kept at a minimum if satisfactory testing is to be accomplished. Such activity results in changes in skin resistance which are difficult to differentiate from galvanic responses to sound. Children with cerebral palsy, particularly of the athetoid type, are usually very difficult to test partly because of the constant involuntary, vermicular movements present. Many of these youngsters also present abnormal psychological patterns secondary to central nervous system damage and/or environmental factors which interfere with PGSR testing. Cerebral palsied youngsters who have severe neuromuscular involvement are difficult to test by conventional techniques and PGSR audiometry, if successful, would be warmly welcomed by those studying these children. The frequent occurrence of bilateral sensorineural hearing impairment in cerebral palsied children, particularly the athetoid group, has been substantiated in a number of reports. (13, 14) These losses of hearing are typically of sufficient severity to interfere with speech and language development, and appropriate audiological management is essential in the total rehabilitation program.

Psychoneurotic and psychotic patients of all ages also prove difficult and, in some cases, impossible to condition for PGSR audiometry. Persons with certain types of endocrine disorders affecting the sweating mechanism are also difficult to condition. Patients with hypothyroidism may fall into this category. The use of infra-red lamps helps induce sweating in some of these patients and may help overcome the problem in some cases.

Emotionally disturbed patients may show marked response to minimal shock stimuli both subjectively and galvanically. These same patients are often not conditionable to auditory stimuli. We have tested some of these patients who fail to show galvanic responses to tone after many tone-shock presentations even at levels where, subjectively, they admit hearing the sound.

Since PGSR testing involves stimulation of the sudoriferous glands, and since the response is believed to be mediated by the autonomic nervous system, patients with a variety of central neuropathologies may prove to be unconditionable. Major medical centers utilizing this technique acknowledge an increasing number of children with communication disorders who are untestable by PGSR audiometry. For the most part, these are the same children who cannot be conditioned by standard techniques. The inability of a child to be conditioned by subjective or galvanic audiometry is generally recognized as evidence of the presence of nonperipheral auditory pathology.

With increased experience with the vagaries of PGSR audiometry clinicians have developed an appreciation of both the advantages and limitations of the technique. The initial enthusiasm and optimism have been tempered by a recognition that PGSR audiometry is not the panacea for the problems of hearing evaluation in children. In the hands of skilled and experienced examiners, it is a valuable addition to the battery of tests available to the paedo-audiologist. Hardy, whose clinical team at Johns Hopkins undoubtedly has amassed more experience with this technique than any other group of clinicians in the world, believes that PGSR testing requires consummate skill.

The pattern of skin resistance varies from individual to individual. The examiner must familiarize himself with the normal skin resistance pattern of each individual tested. The decision as to whether a given galvanic response represents a true reaction to the auditory stimulus or whether it has occurred in association with a nonauditory stimulus is often not easy to reach. Physical movements or emotional reactions and distractions occurring during the test affect the patient's responses and make the interpretation of test responses very difficult. Because of the many subjective factors involved in the examiner's interpretation of galvanic responses, Goodhill (15) and his associates feel that PGSR audiometry is not by any means an objective technique and that the search for a truly objective method of audiometry must be continued. The use of the acoustic impedance meter, when properly calibrated and clinically evaluated, may prove to be such a technique.

In one version of this technique, (16) one ear is used as an indicator ear and the intra-tympanic muscle reflexes are measured by changes in tension of the tympanic membrane with the impedance meter while the other ear is tested with a succession of sound intensities to establish the reflex threshold. The level at which the muscle reflex is elicited is compared with the threshold for pure tones. The difference between these thresholds is smaller in the patient with a cochlear lesion than in patients with nonrecruting hearing losses. This instrument, is also believed to be of value in the detection of nonorganic hearing impairments and differentiating among such conditions as ossicular chain discontinuities, congenital aplasias and ageneses of the ossicles and otosclerosis. An improved impedance bridge for clinical use developed by Drs. Zwislocki and Feldman of Syracuse University is now commercially available.

PGSR audiometry using speech rather than pure tones as the stimulus has been used in evaluating the hearing of adults with suspected nonorganic hearing impairments. Ruhm and Menzel (17) devised a test based upon differential conditioning to a key word selected from a list of conventional spondee words. PGSR audiometry using speech material as the stimulus has not been applied to the testing of children but appears worthy of investigation. Its use with children would be limited to those with adequate language comprehension. Retardation or absence of speech would not present a problem since the child is not asked to give an overt response to the material presented. However, adequate language comprehension is required. The relation of hearing for speech and for pure tones might be established in some children by the use of PGSR audiometry to determine thresholds for each type of stimulus. If, as has been claimed, a selective deafness for pure tones exists in some children, the speech PGSR test might help to establish valid thresholds for such children. Lists of specially prepared spondee words for children have been prepared by Utley (18) and could serve as the test material for the development of a speech PGSR test for children.

In summary, PGSR audiometry when properly utilized as part of a total diagnostic work-up, including a careful and detailed history, can yield valuable information about the child's auditory function. Its assets, as well as its limitations, should be fully appreciated.

ELECTROENCEPHALOGRAPHIC AUDIOMETRY

A relatively new approach to electrophysiological audiometry involves the use of the electroencephalogram (EEG) to record responses to auditory stimuli. Several institutions are now actively engaged in research on this technique. The results thus far have suggested considerable potential for the use of this method with children. EEG audiometry is not yet a standard clinical procedure and must at present be considered to be in the experimental stage.

The brain continually generates electrical potentials whether the patient is awake or asleep. Unlike PGSR responses which tend to be suppressed when the patient is sedated or asleep, electroencephalographic audiometry (EEGA[1]) can be successfully performed on a sleeping or sedated patient. This enables the audiologist to apply this technique to children who are so hyperactive, motor disinhibited, or emotionally disturbed, that they cannot be evaluated unless they are adequately sedated.

A pediatric neurologist and an experienced, well-trained EEG technician are important members of the team evaluating the hearing of children by this technique. The child should be mildly sedated during EEGA. Because many of the children requiring evaluation by this technique may have central nervous system (CNS) damage which has not been conclusively established at the time of the test, the choice of sedation must be made with great care. The pediatric neurologist, in consultation with an anesthesiologist should explore this problem and decide upon a suitable agent for the particular patient.

---

[1]The abbreviations EEA and EER have been used for electroencephalographic audiometry and electroencephalographic response by some authors. Since the contraction EEG has become an almost universally accepted abbreviation for the electroencephalogram the authors feel that the terms EEGA and EEGR would serve better than EEA and EER to designate electroencephalographic audiometry and electroencephalographic response respectively, and we have so used them in this text.

With the child mildly sedated and lightly asleep, the EEGA pattern shows a change from the "sleeping" to the "waking" pattern in response to auditory stimuli which have been "heard." The "arousal" response is considered evidence of the patient's having heard the sound presented.

A problem discussed in connection with PGSR audiometry was galvanic responses to nonauditory stimuli, both physiological and psychological. This problem also affects EEGA. Many nonauditory stimuli, both internal and external, are capable of producing an arousal response. Futhermore, persons do not give electroencephalographic responses (EEGR) to all sounds presented even though they may be of sufficient intensity to arouse a response under other conditions. Adaptation to auditory stimuli occurs in EEGA as with PGSR and the more often a sound is presented, the less likely it is to evoke a response. Still another complicating factor is that the EEG pattern itself (i.e., no auditory stimulus) may change while the patient is asleep and it becomes enormously difficult to differentiate responses to auditory stimuli from spontaneous changes in the EEG record.

EEGA has, however, several important advantages over PGSR audiometry which are of sufficient magnitude to justify continuing interest in the technique in spite of the difficulties present. PGSR testing is relatively unsuccessful in evaluating the hearing of children below eighteen months of age. The normal skin resistance of such children is generally very high and it becomes very difficult to demonstrate changes in skin resistance during the test. EEGA has been quite successful in this age group.

PGSR responses are affected by the use of sedation. Withrow and Goldstein (19) have tested many young children successfully by EEGA while these children were asleep. Apparently, mild sedation to induce sleep does not reduce EEGA responsiveness. Many children we are called upon to evaluate have severe neurological and psychological abnormalities which make a hearing evaluation without the use of adequate sedation difficult or impossible. Children with severe cerebral palsy, "brain-damaged" children exhibiting the Strauss-Lehtinen syndrome, (20) and autistic children often fall into this category. To elicit meaningful diagnostic information on the hearing of such children requires the use of a test modality which is unaffected by the use of sufficient sedation to place the patient in a relaxed, manageable state for the duration of the test. EEGA offers the promise of solving this important problem.

It is important to emphasize the present experimental nature of EEGA. Although this approach is promising and potentially capable of becoming one of our most valuable tools in auditory assessment of young children, standardization of the test technique and the interpretation of responses have not reached a point where the method is applicable to routine clinical use.

Two groups of workers have pioneered in the development of EEGA. One group is headed by Dr. Robert Goldstein of the Jewish Hospital and the Central Institute for the Deaf in St. Louis. The second group is led by Dr. A. J. Derbyshire of the Harper Hospital of Detroit, the Parmly Foundation for Auditory Research and the Illinois Institute for Technology in Chicago. These two groups of workers have cooperated in several phases of research. However, there are still major differences between the two groups on a number of fundamental aspects of EEGA particularly with regard to the interpretation of test response patterns.

Derbyshire and his associates (21) used a barbiturate for sedation of their patients who ranged in age from three months to two years and seven months. They used a Grass eight-channel electroencephalograph in conjunction with a standard pure tone audiometer. The eight electrodes were attached to the right and left frontal, parietal, occipital and temporal areas of the cranium. The four types of responses noted were: an "on" effect, usually a K-complex pattern; a continuous effect; an "off" effect; and a delayed reaction. These four types of responses have also been described by Goldstein and his associates in several studies which have appeared in the literature. Derbyshire and associates in the reference previously cited found that EEGA thresholds in twenty-two patients were in agreement with conventional audiometric thresholds within a range of plus or minus 18 db. They believe these EEGRs are associated with some "simple" type of CNS arousal mechanism. This is based upon the diffuseness of response, lack of influence of age on response in the age group employed in their study, and the ability of the response to be duplicated in other sensory modalities. The controlled variants in the test situation which affect the response are the depth of sedation-induced sleep, the quantity and type of sedation administered, variation in stimulus-presentation patterns, and mid-test shifts in procedure. Derbyshire and his co-workers consider EEGA clinically useful when combined with other available data. EEGA in their opinion should *not* be used as the sole basis for arriving at a conclusion as to the nature of the communication disorder present.

Derbyshire believes that EEGA complements rather than replaces other forms of audiometric examination. Although he considers it useful as an independent assessor of hearing function, it is better employed as a complement to other audiometric procedures by providing information from another level of the auditory pathway. He further suggests that the differentiated results of standard subjective audiometry, PGSR audiometry and EEGA when compared on a single patient present a composite picture of the available amounts of audiological information at each of several levels in the auditory transmissive system, i.e., perceptive, reflexive and cortical levels. Furehermore, the combined use of all these methods may yield an objective distinction regarding the locus of auditory deficit. (22) Eventually, other types of audiometric tests may be developed which will give still more definitive information on the site(s) of lesion contributing to the child's auditory pathology.

Derbyshire and Farley believe that there are two principal problems involved in the development of EEGA for clinical purposes: the degree of interpretive skill required, and the need for standardization of test and interpretive procedures. They believe that a complete understanding of all brain wave patterns is not necessary in utilizing this procedure for hearing evaluation. Rather, the interpreter of EEGA must master *only* several patterns of changes which have been found to accompany auditory stimulation, e.g., voltage increases and decreases, K-complex formations, spindles, alpha or Berger 5-7 per second interruptions. The EEG record is then correlated with the auditory stimulus. To resolve the second problem, Derbyshire and his co-workers (21, 22, 23) have suggested several methods for validation of EEGA results. First was the use of appropriate statistical procedures to establish "cortical auditory thresholds." More recently, they have suggested an improved method of analysis of cortical response to tone by the measurement of shifts in the brain wave pattern recorded simultaneously with the auditory stimulus. This recording of pattern changes is later analyzed for indications of receptions of the tones presented. An electronic recorder is used in conjunction with a standard polygraph. The cortex has indicated a response when the recorder produces a shift in frequency. This shift occurs within a specified time interval after the presentation of the tone.

Charan and Goldstein (24) also emphasize the importance of using more than one method of assessing hearing in children. They believe that the combined use of EEGA and PGSR is clinically desirable whenever possible. Of the two forms of electrophysiological audiometry, Goldstein considers EEGA the more valuable clinically, and the one he would prefer to use if forced to limit himself to one method of evaluation on a given patient. He has been able successfully to test infants and very young children by EEGA. Although both EEGA and PGSR audiometry are affected by adaptation, in Goldstein's experience EEGA is less subject to both adaptation and extinction than PGSR.

Withrow and Goldstein (20) list the following advantages of EEGA over PGSR: No conditioning is necessary with EEGA. In PGSR testing, the child often squirms because of the shock, the wires or boredom. In EEGA, these problems are resolved since testing is performed while the child is asleep. Goldstein and his associates believe, however, that it is considerably *more* difficult to interpret EEGR than PGSR responses. Furthermore, no overt responses to sound are possible when the patient is asleep so that no correlation is possible between subjective and electrophysiological responses.

Goldstein *et al.* have found that when EEGA and PGSR tests are combined, the results yield an estimate of hearing within plus or minus 10 db. of the subjective threshold. When only one test can be administered, the EEGA is preferred by them. Goldstein and Derbyshire both agree that whenever possible results of *both* types of test should be utilized, and combined with other forms of audiometric examination.

REFERENCES

(1) Davis, H. and Silverman, S. R., eds.: *Hearing and Deafness.* Rev. ed., Holt, Rinehart and Winston, New York, 1960, p. 231; p. 482.

(2) Hirsh, I. J.: *The Measurement of Hearing.* McGraw-Hill Book Co., New York, 1952, p. 264.

(3) Hardy, W. G. and Bordley, J. E.: Special techniques in testing the hearing of children. *J. Speech and Hearing Disorders, 16*:122, (June) 1951.

(4) Hardy, W. G. and Pauls, M. D.: The test situation in PGSR audiometry. *J. Speech and Hearing Disorders, 17*:13, (March) 1952.

(5) Richter, C. P.: The electrical skin resistance; diurnal and daily variations in psychopathic and in normal persons. *Arch. Neurol. and Psychiat., 19*:488, (March) 1928.

(6) Richter, C. P.: Physiological factors involved in the electrical resistance of the skin. *Am. J. Physiol., 88*:596, (May) 1929.

(7) Richter, C. P.: The sweat glands studied by the electrical resistance method. *Am. J. Physiol., 68*:147, (March) 1924.

(8) Richter, C. P. and Whelan, F. G.: Description of a skin galvanometer that gives a graphic record of activity in the sympathetic nervous system. *J. Neurosurg, 6*:279, (July) 1949.

(9) Bordley, J. E.: An evaluation of the psychogalvanic skin-resistance technique in audiometry. *Laryngoscope, 66*:1162, (Sept.) 1956.

(10) Bordley, J. E. and Haskins, H. L.: The role of the cerebrum in hearing. *Ann. Otol., Rhin. and Laryng., 64*:370, (June) 1955.

(11) Haskins, H. L.: Differential diagnosis of hearing problems of adult patients. *Laryngoscope, 66*:658, (June) 1956.

(12) Portmann, M. and Portmann, G.: The place of objective audiometry in the functional study of the young deaf. *Voix du Silence, 4*:12, 1960.

(13) Zaner, A. and Miller, M. H.: Hearing problems in athetoid cerebral palsy: preliminary report of case findings. *A.M.A. Arch. Otolaryng., 70*:776, (Dec.) 1959.

(14) Fisch, L.: Deafness in cerebral-palsied school-children. *Lancet, 2*:370, (Aug. 20) 1955.

(15) Goodhill, V., Rehman, I. and Brockman, S. J.: Objective skin resistance audiometry: the electro-audiogram. *Ann. Otol., Rhin. and Laryng., 63*:22, (March) 1954.

(16) Madsen Electronics Co., Madsen acoustic impedance meter; general information and operating instructions.

(17) Ruhm, H. B. and Menzel, O. J.: Objective speech audiometry in cases of nonorganic hearing loss. *A.M.A. Arch. Otolaryng.,* *69*:212, (Feb.) 1959.

(18) Utley, J.: *What's Its Name?*: A Guide to Speech and Hearing Development. Univ. of Ill. Press, Urbana, 1951, p. 126.

(19) Withrow, F. B., Jr. and Goldstein, R.: An electrophysiologic procedure for determination of auditory threshold in children. *Laryngoscope, 68*:1674, (Sept.) 1958.

(20) Strauss, A. A. and Lehtinen, L. E.: *Psychopathology and Education of the Brain-Injured Child.* Grune and Stratton, New York, 1947.

(21) Derbyshire, A. J. et al: Audiometric measurements by electroencephalography. *Electroencephalog. and Clin. Neurophysiol., 8*:467, (Aug.) 1956.

(22) Derbyshire, A. J. and Farley, J. C.: Sampling auditory responses at the cortical level: a routine for EEG audiometric testing. *Ann. Otol., Rhin. and Laryng., 68*:675, (Sept.) 1959.

(23) Norkus, F. J. et al: Frequency measure of the EEG. *J. Acous. Soc. Amer., 32*:1147, 1960.

(24) Charan, K. K. and Goldstein, R.: Relation between the EEG pattern and the ease of eliciting electrodermal responses. *J. Speech and Hearing Disorders, 22*:651, (Dec.) 1957.

Chapter V

DIAGNOSTIC AND THERAPEUTIC PROBLEMS IN THE TOTAL MANAGEMENT OF CHILDREN WITH AUDITORY DISORDERS

In this chapter, a series of youngsters will be described who present problems requiring the use of one or more of the test procedures which have been considered thus far. These children have been selected from among the more than 3,000 patients referred to the Hearing and Speech Clinic of Kings County Hospital Center[1] in Brooklyn, New York since its opening in June, 1959. They are illustrative of some of the challenging diagnostic and therapeutic problems encountered in a major municipal hospital. These patients also illustrate the necessity of a "team" approach to the evaluation of communication disorders and of the need for a close and continuing liaison with other agencies in the community, both medical and educational.

Each of these children received a routine medical evaluation consisting of a pediatric and otolaryngologic examination. They were then evaluated by the other members of the Hearing and Speech Clinic staff who performed audiological, speech and language, psychological and social evaluations. When indicated, specialized examinations were also performed which included pediatric neurology and psychiatry, serological studies and X-Ray examinations.

PATIENT I. M.J., Male, Born 9/21/49. *Failure to detect profound, bilateral deafness until age 12 in a child with congenitally deaf parents.*

---

[1]This facility functions as part of the Division of Otolaryngology of the State University of New York Downstate Medical Center, and is fully approved under the Hearing Conservation Program of the Bureau for Handicapped Children of the City of New York Department of Health. The organization, objectives and philosophy of this program are described in detail in the Appendix.

[65]

This patient was referred by another institution in the area with a request for a neurological examination including EEG and a psychological evaluation. The impression of the referring agency was that the child's lack of speech and language development was secondary to aphasia and possible mental retardation. Hearing was judged to be "normal or near normal."

Both of the boy's parents have been profoundly deaf since birth. The delivery was normal and full term. General motor development was within normal limits. At the age of five, a colloid goiter was found and he was treated with iodine and thyroid extract with resulting decrease in the size of the thyroid gland. His father reported that the patient had a habit of rocking his head before going to sleep and that he frequently laughed for no apparent reason.

When the patient was first seen in the Hearing and Speech Clinic, he was attending a class for children with retarded mental development in a public school. He had previously been placed in a class for aphasic children in a school for the deaf but was reassigned when school authorities decided his main problem was mental retardation. He had also received one year of speech therapy at one of the local speech and hearing centers but was discharged because he had made little or no progress.

The pediatric and otologic examinations were negative except for a small, movable nodule in the left lobe of the thyroid gland, and the speech and language retardation. No intra or extracranial lesions were demonstrable on skull x-rays. Neurological examination and EEG were also normal.

Speech and language development were severely retarded. The patient was able to produce only a few monosyllabic words which were largely unintelligible even to members of his family. Interview with the grandmother revealed that no words at all were spoken until the age of six years. At the time of the evaluation speech comprehension was extremely limited. The overall voice pattern was monotonous and without inflection.

Performance tests of intelligence only could be administered by the Hearing and Speech Clinic psychologist. Verbal tests could not be utilized. The patient had an I.Q. of 48 on the performance scale of the Wechsler Intelligence Scale for Children (WISC). A score of under 50 was obtained on the Chicago Non-Verbal examination. It was felt from a *qualitative* analysis of the results of these tests that the patient's inherent intellectual capacities were higher than was reflected by the I.Q. scores. This was inferred from his performance on the block design and coding subtests of the WISC and the transposing of symbols into numbers on the Chicago test both of which were considerably better than his performance on all other sub-tests.

The patient showed very limited intellectual and motor development by the distorted and perseverative quality of his Bender-Gestalt reproductions. His human figure drawings were extremely immature and suggested the productions of a much younger child.

The patient's pure tone audiometric thresholds were determined without difficulty and the pure tone audiogram shown in in Figure 5 was obtained. This audiogram shows the presence of a profound, bilateral loss of hearing of the sensorineural type. The loss of hearing for the "speech frequency range" (500, 1000 and 2000 sps) averages 93 plus db. in the right ear and 83 db. in the left. No responses could be elicited to bone conduction stimuli. There was no measurable hearing within audiometric limits above 1000 cps in the right ear and above 2000 cps in the left.

This patient now functions on an extremely retarded level in

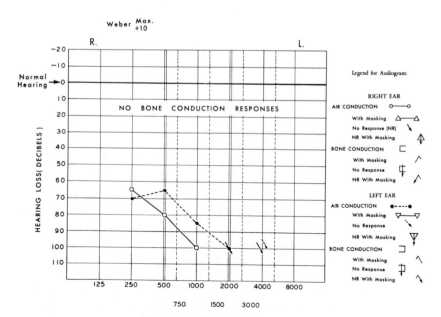

Fig. 5. Audiogram. Patient I.

all areas and the prognosis is very unfavorable. Although he had been evaluated on a "piece-meal" basis since the age of five, the diagnosis of profound, bilateral sensorineural deafness was not made until December, 1961 when he was twelve years of age. High gain, high power amplification and an intensive program of hearing and speech therapy should have been instituted many years ago. The deafness of the boy's parents further contributed to the problem since they communicate primarily through sign language and could provide little or no speech and language stimulation in the home. Much valuable time had been lost and proper audiological management at this late date cannot compensate for the failure to detect this problem in time and to have instituted an appropriate rehabilitation program.

PATIENT II. C.C., Male, Born 10/10/58. *Complex problem of differential diagnosis in a 3 year old emotionally disturbed boy.*

The patient was born in October, 1958 following a normal full term gestation. Delivery was normal. Discharge from the right ear of two to three weeks duration occurred at two months of age and was treated successfully with antibiotics. He had been subject since that episode to a number of attacks of suppurative otitis media, primarily affecting the right ear. Early in 1960, the boy's parents noticed that his speech development "came to a halt" and he seemed to ignore spoken words. His parents reported that he responded only to loud TV commercials. A private otolaryngologist examined the patient in August, 1960, suspected that a significant hearing loss seemed to be present, and referred the child to the Hearing and Speech Clinic for complete evaluation. He was first seen in the Clinic in September 1960 at which time the family was residing in a neighboring state. A preliminary sound field evaluation suggested the possibility of a hearing loss and observation of the child's behavior suggested emotional problems. It was decided that it would be more convenient for the family to have the evaluation completed by an agency closer to their place of residence since there was obviously a problem present which required extended work with the child. In January, 1961, adenotonsillectomy was performed because of recurrent episodes of suppurative otitis media and the presence of enlarged tonsils and adenoids. Bilateral myringotomies were performed at the time of surgery and a "thick, milky white fluid" was removed from each ear.

Having moved back to Brooklyn, the patient was re-evaluated by our Clinic Pediatrician in March, 1962, at three and one-half years of age. Physical examination was within normal limits. A complete bloodcount and skull x-rays were normal. On otological examination both external auditory canals were normal. Both ear drums were found to be dull and slightly hyperemic. Hypertrophied lymphoid tissue on the posterior pharyngeal wall was noted. Small lymph nodes were present bilaterally in the neck. The examining otologist noted extreme restlessness and hyperactivity of the child.

Subsequent to the above medical examinations, a number of attempts were made to assess the status of the child's hearing. The everpresent hyperactivity made hearing evaluation difficult. He could not be trained to give any kind of repeatable response to pure tone stimuli on the first or subsequent hearing evaluation sessions. He was scheduled for a series of play-conditioning training sessions but these were also unsuccessful. Observation of the child's auditory behavior and sound field responses to a variety of sound stimuli led us to conclude that the boy's hearing was within normal limits and unrelated to the communication problem present.

A speech and language evaluation was attempted with little success. It appeared at the time of the evaluation that the child had developed very limited language and had three or four words in his vocabulary apparently intelligible only to his parents. His vocalizations consisted primarily of babbling. He appeared to have relatively normal inflectional patterns during the babbling. He was extremely uncooperative during the evaluation and refused to participate in any activities proposed by the examiner. His mother reported that in order to communicate with others, the patient pulled the person to the object he desired.

Several psychological examinations were performed on this yougster. The initial psychological evaluation done in September, 1960, at age two years, indicated that, intellectually, the child was functioning on the average to bright-normal level of intelligence. The Vineland Social Maturity Scale was administered to the mother and the Stanford-Binet Intelligence Scale and Gesell Developmental Schedules were administered to the child. Evidence of emotional disturbance was noted in the child's hyperactive, restless behavior during the examination and the psychologist recommended that he be referred to the Child Guidance Clinic for further evaluation by a pediatric psychiatrist. The most recent psychological evaluation was performed in February, 1962. His age at the time of that test was three years and four months. The psychologist found that testing the child was virtually impossible as he became increasingly restless and uncontrollable during the examination. When the psychologist attempted to exercise some control over his physical activity he would fall to the floor and begin rolling about like an infant while holding the examiner's hand. His mother described similar behavior at home. She also reported no success in her attempts at toilet training the child.

On this psychological evaluation no formal I.Q. could be obtained. Qualitative analysis of his few test responses supported the previous finding of normal intelligence. His extreme shifts in behavior, hyperactivity, short attention span and restlessness suggested either emotional disturbance, or central nervous system involvement, or a combination of both. An evaluation was performed in March, 1962, in the Pediatric Neurology Clinic. The neurologist considered the patient's basic problem to be emotional rather than organic, possibly one of the childhood schizophrenias. He placed the youngster on Dextro-Amphetamine Sulfate, 2.5 mg., twice daily and suggested an evaluation by the Child Psychiatry Clinic.

The patient was seen in the Child Psychiatric Clinic in May, 1962. It was the impression of the psychiatrist that the diagnosis of schizophrenia was not justified, although some degree of emotional disturbance was definitely present.

The patient has been receiving individual speech and hearing therapy once weekly in the Hearing and Speech Clinic since February, 1962. It was found that the child functions best in a highly-structured therapy situation having a minimum of distractions. Our therapist now finds that a more permissive attitude is increasingly possible and the patient is now allowed to select his own play activities during the therapy session. The objectives of the therapy program are to stimulate increased speech and language development, improve general behavior and increase the ability of the child to work with others, both children and adults. He has begun to use single words such as "car," "cow," "hat," and "milk" and short phrases meaningfully. His comprehension of speech appears to be normal for his age. Although the therapy program has been administered in a structured situation, little direct or formal speech and hearing therapy has been used.

The present, tentative working diagnosis is that this patient's communication disorder is secondary to emotional disturbance and possible minimal central nervous system deficit manifested primarily by bizarre behavior. It is our impression at this time that the boy is not "aphasic" in the usual sense although some degree of expressive aphasia remains a possibility. We believe he requires an intensive program of rehabilitation and the opportunity to socialize with other children. We have recommended that he be referred to the Day Treatment Center of a local agency. This agency is associated with the Division of Pediatric Psychiatry of a large general hospital. The agency offers a nursery school for the treatment of educable children three to six years of age suffering from behavior disorders or emotional problems. It also provides counseling services for the parents of such children. It is our feeling that such placement will significantly contribute to further progress and improvement in a number of areas. The speech and hearing therapy sessions at our Clinic will be continued while the child attends the Day Treatment Center.

The definitive diagnosis of this child's communication problem must await his response to further rehabilitation and special education.

PATIENT III. H.B.E., Female, Born 10/25/57. *Excellent response to amplification in a child with profound, bilateral deafness.*

This child was referred with a chief complaint of absence of speech development. Our initial evaluation was performed at age two and one-half years. She was born following a normal, full term pregnancy. Labor lasted nineteen hours. Following delivery she did not cry for four minutes. The developmental history was within normal limits: held head erect at five months, sat unsupported at eight months, walked alone at thirteen months. She babbled a great deal as an infant. According to the mother, the patient was able to understand almost all of what was said to her. It was noted that the mother's speech was highly animated and accompanied by many gestures and facial expressions.

The pediatric examination was normal. Otologic examination revealed minimal scarring of the tympanic membranes and moderately enlarged tonsils and adenoids. It was noted during the examination that the child had no gag reflex, even during indirect laryngoscopic examination. A subsequent neurological examination, suggested because of the absence of the gag reflex, was otherwise entirely normal.

The child's speech did not progress beyond the babbling stage. When seen at the age of two and one-half for a speech and language evaluation, she communicated by pointing, gesturing and leading the individual to a particular object.

Results of a psychological evaluation in which the Vineland Social Maturity Scale was administered to the mother and performance items of the Stanford-Binet to the child indicated that intellectual function was on the near normal to normal level.

When first evaluated audiologically, the patient did not respond to any auditory stimuli presented to her at the maximum level of the equipment used. On PGSR testing, the child could not be conditioned to any pure tone at the maximum levels possible with the equipment. There was considerable response to the shock stimulus but conditioning to the pure tone stimulus could not be accomplished.

The child was placed on a program of regular, individual auditory training with trial use of high gain, high power amplification. After six months of intensive training supplemented by supportive work at home, she responded at 500 cps to a level of 95 db. re: audiometric zero. As therapy continued, which included

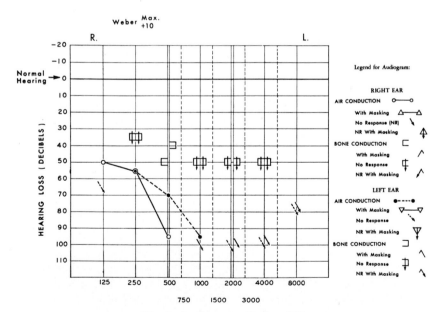

Fig. 6. Audiogram. Patient III.

intensive training in responding to auditory stimuli, reliable responses at other frequencies were elicited and a pure tone audiogram was established which is shown in Figure 6. It was felt that it was not the child's hearing which changed during the six month period but, rather, her ability to attend and respond consistently to auditory stimuli. The fact that she was six months older also helped considerably. It is important to note in terms of parent counseling by the physician that we were unable to assess reliably the status of this child's hearing until a six month period of intensive auditory training had been completed. The audiogram reveals a profound, near total, loss of hearing, but residual hearing is definitely present in both ears in the lower portion of the "speech frequency range."

A series of high gain, high power hearing aids were tried and loaned to the patient following a period of two months during which an auditory training unit utilizing automatic-gain-control was used during the therapy sessions. Automatic-gain-control or compression amplification is a method of limiting the maximum power handling capacity of an amplifying system to a level below the threshold of discomfort of the user. Sounds above this level are almost instantaneously fed back to a lower stage of amplification. The advantage of this system of output control is that the wave form is less distorted than it is when the more frequently used system of symmetrical peak clipping is employed. A study by Lynn and Carhart (1) indicates that patients with endolymphatic hydrops and presbyacusis achieve improved discrimination scores when the system of compression amplification incorporates a release time of under 400 ms. Release time refers to the interval between the instant when the input signal drops and the moment when the gain has risen sufficiently to become established at the proper level.

The distinguishing feature of compression amplifiers is that a change in the level of the input signal modifies the gain of the system reducing the necessity of frequent adjustments by the user of the instrument's gain control. A number of auditory training units, some conventionally worn hearing aids and at least one "ear level" hearing aid employ some form of compression amplification. This feature was found particularly advantageous with this patient who had a marked narrowing of the dynamic range, i.e., the difference between the threshold of hearing and the threshold of discomfort.

Four conventionally worn aids were loaned to the patient for a period of one month each and the parents were given training in helping the child use the hearing aids at home and in observing the child's responses to amplification under different conditions. Reports of the child's responses with each of the aids were made by the parents to the therapist. These reports were added to the results of a sound field hearing aid evaluation to enable the clinician to reach a final decision on which aid was to be recommended for this patient. Figure 7 shows the gain at threshold which is provided by this hearing aid. Testing was performed with frequency modulated pure tones in a sound field with and without the hearing aid. In spite of the profound loss of hearing present, this patient obtains an improvement of 45 db. at 500 cps and 50 db. at 1000 cps. Without an aid, the child did not hear 2000 and 4000 cps at the maximum level possible with

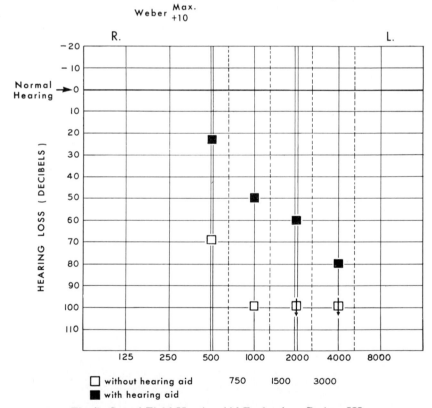

Fig. 7. Sound Field Hearing Aid Evaluation. Patient III.

the instrumentation used. With amplification, her thresholds are 60 and 80 db. respectively at these frequencies, representing a gain of at least 40 and 20 db.

Standard speech audiometry could not be used to evaluate this child's response to amplification because of her limited vocabulary and poor speech intelligibility. Whenever possible, of course, speech audiometry is the method of choice for evaluating performance with amplification since speech represents the functional stimulus the child will be called upon to hear in actual listening situations. Futhermore, it is important to ascertain performance at levels above threshold since few sounds in every day life are at or near threshold levels.

The severity of this child's hearing loss and her response to auditory rehabilitation thus far indicate the need for placement in a school for the deaf, which is now being arranged. However, the early detection of this problem, the intensive program of auditory rehabilitation which has been instituted, and the excellent response to amplification indicate a favorable prognosis. This child can, with the continuation of intensive auditory rehabilitation, including speech reading and speech therapy, be expected to develop fully intelligible (although not normal) speech and to function adequately in all social and vocational situations.

PATIENT IV. T.L., Female, Born 6/9/59. *Profound bilateral hearing loss in child with no other contributory factors.*

This child was delivered with forceps following a pregnancy which was normal except for "staining" during the first weeks after conception. The parents observed lack of response to sounds of soft and moderate intensity when the child was about two and one-half years of age.

The pediatric and otologic examinations were within normal limits. A series of play-conditioning sessions were arranged in which the child was trained to give a consistent response to pure tone stimuli. By the age of three, a complete pure tone air and bone conduction audiogram had been performed which was considered reliable and valid by the examiners. This audiogram is shown in Figure 8. The child has a profound loss of hearing which averages 80 db. in the right ear and 85 db. in the left for the "speech frequency range." There is residual hearing present throughout this range in both ears. The loss is primarily of the

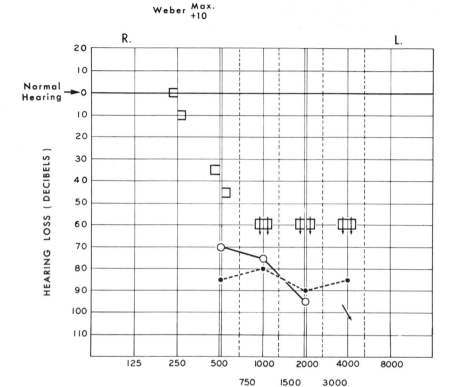

Fig. 8. Audiogram. Patient IV.

sensorineural type with a possible conductive component in the low frequencies.

When first evaluated by the speech pathologist, the child demonstrated no meaningful speech. A series of high pitched squeals constituted her only vocalizations. Communication with others was made through animated gestures accompanied by vivid facial expressions.

The results of the psychological evaluation indicated a friendly, well-adjusted child whose intellectual capacities fell well within the normal range.

This patient has been enrolled in an intensive program of auditory rehabilitation in which she has made excellent progress. She has been assisted by extremely cooperative parents who have made an excellent adjustment to the child's handicap. Binaural amplification has been successfully used throughout the training program both in the Clinic and at home. A series of binaural, conventionally worn aids have been loaned to the family, and the child's responses to them have been observed carefully by the parents and reported to the hearing therapist. Following the four month trial period, a binaural aid was selected and recommended for full time use. The child now uses the aid from early morning to bed time. When she dresses herself in the morning, her hearing aids are put on and dressing is not considered complete without them. Her speech development has improved tremendously during the period that she has been with us. Her vocabulary has grown steadily and she is now undergoing rapid speech and language development.

She has been placed in a regular nursery school where she is getting along very well. Amplification is used throughout the day at school and is well accepted by the other children and teachers. This child will be enrolled in a regular public school with normal hearing youngsters. She will require many years of intensive auditory rehabilitation. With such assistance and appropriate and continued counseling of the parents, she can be expected to achieve a satisfactory and satisfying adjustment in a normal hearing environment.

PATIENT V. O.J., Male, Born 9/4/55. *Inability to establish conclusive diagnosis in child with severe communication and behavior disorder.*

This child was referred in 1961 at age five and one-half years by the Speech and Hearing Clinic of a large voluntary medical center in the New York City area. He had been referred to their Speech and Hearing Clinic in October, 1957, by their Pediatrics Department with an impression of "retarded development of speech and locomotion and bilateral marked hearing loss." During the period in which he was evaluated at their Speech and Hearing Clinic, he had several episodes of discharging ears. His tonsils and adenoids were removed in March, 1958. A hearing test performed in December, 1960, showed an everage loss of 30 db. bilaterally. Their final impression was that the child was mainly retarded and that the mild hearing loss was aggravating but not causing his generally poor development.

When we first saw this child he was attending a parochial school for the deaf where he was doing very poorly. His disruptive classroom behavior was making him increasingly unmanageable.

An otological examination was performed in March, 1961. The child appeared frightened and cried throughout the examination. The otologic findings were essentially normal. The pediatrician noted that the youngster had had measles at two years of age with fever as high as 105° for several days. Two siblings, one older and one younger, have known sensorineural hearing losses since birth. There is no history of Rh incompatability or viral disease during pregnancy. The child was born weighing 8 pounds, 4 ounces, following a full-term, normal pregnancy and delivery.

This patient was not affectionate, related poorly to others and always played alone. There was no history of trauma, convulsions or loss of consciousness. He had never spoken words, but was able to cry and shout when angry.

A psychological examination was performed one month later. Qualitative analysis of responses to the performance items of the Stanford-Binet Intelligence Test indicated that the boy was functioning on the borderline level of intelligence. He demonstrated such signs as short attention span, distractability and motor disinhibition strongly suggestive of a central nervous system deficit. During the speech and language evaluation, the patient demonstrated no speech. His mother reported to the examiner that he had frequent temper tantrums at home and seemed to enjoy breaking things. He used to grind his teeth and later made cracking noises with his mouth. His mother stated that he seemed to be "in another world" and she was unable to cope with his behavior.

He was first evaluated audiologically in April, 1961. It was the impression of the examiners that the youngster had a possible mild hearing loss. It was further their impression that problems other than hearing loss were more significant contributing factors to the lack of speech and language development and the behavior problem. Further audiological evaluation supported this impression. Even though this youngster is now almost seven years of age, we have still been unable to condition him to respond to a pure tone audiometric test. We are still forced to rely on observation of his responses to auditory stimuli presented in a sound field. PGSR testing has been attempted but the child's behavior was such that he would not permit the examiners to attach the electrodes to him.

Neurological examination by observation only revealed no evidence of spasticity, impairment of gait, ataxia, nystagmus or impaired coordination.

In spite of the essentially negative neurological findings, it is our feeling that this youngster's communication and behavior disorder is related, at least in part, to a central nervous system deficit not sufficiently gross to show up on present neurological test procedures. Our case worker visited the school for the deaf which the patient was attending and learned that his behavior was completely uncontrollable. According to the teacher in charge, he did not participate in any way in any of the group activities and had been unable to relate in any way either to them or to the children. His behavior was perseverative and impulsive. He ran around the room most of the time and did whatever he felt like doing. He did not seem to be interested in any activity involving new learning of any kind. He often adopted unusual positions and seemed to find comfort in them. For example, he enjoyed lying with his head on the floor and his legs on his teacher's lap. His teacher indicated that at times he remained in these positions for hours at a time and appeared to be quite content. In spite of his compulsive behavior, he did not seem to be either an aggressive or hostile child. He would react negatively to attempts by others to control his behavior but otherwise would remain by himself and seem quite content. He did not appear to be benefitting to any degree from the educational program of the school.

A recommendation was made that the child be admitted to a class for aphasic children in the public school. He was evaluated by the school psychiatrist in March, 1962. Upon entering the psychiatrist's office, he began to run around and push the furniture. Every contact with the psychiatrist was avoided and rejected even to the extent of pushing back toys, paper, pencils, etc. After forty-five minutes in which the parents talked to the psychiatrist, he hesitatingly explored the possibility of reaching for the glove puppets which he spied on the table. Mobilizing sufficent spontaneous freedom to reach out and get them required another fifteen minutes. He appeared to derive pleasure from physical activity. There was also evident an active interest in making music, combining the puppets, the horn and the accordion. As he became acclimated to the situation, he demonstrated a progressive capacity for invention and exploration of the situation and the objects. He enjoyed building a tottering tower with the blocks, then crashed it down, showing interest in the results of his action. He evidenced more interest in objects than in people throughout the visit. The impression of the school psychiatrist was that the patient had: (1) a mixed receptive and expressive aphasia; (2) congenital and developmental central nervous system damage; and (3) a bilateral hearing loss. He has been admitted to the public school aphasia program.

This child demonstrates retarded speech and language development and severe behavioral disturbances secondary to central nervous system involvement. This diagnosis is made in spite of the negative findings on standard neurological examinations and the absence of a history of seizures, trauma or accident. The psychological disturbances are secondary to the neurological deficit and no primary childhood psychosis is present. A hearing loss of still undetermined degree and type may contribute to the problem. His progress will be followed in the aphasia program and he will be recalled to the Hearing and Speech Clinic regularly for complete re-evaluation. The final complete diagnosis must await observation of his response to the special educational regimen and further development and maturation.

PATIENT VI. R.L.G., Male, Born 6/6/49. *Nonorganic hearing loss in a 13 year old with many psychosomatic complaints.*

This patient has a history of chronic gastronintestinal disorder on a functional basis treated on an ambulatory basis over a six year period. Complaints include perianal itching, chronic constipation and abdominal pain. All tests including a complete gastro-intestinal x-ray series, stool cultures, and parasite ova workup were entirely negative. A pediatrician felt, after examining this patient during one of his many visits to the hospital that most of his complaints reflected a lack of "tender loving care" and a search for attention.

In February, 1960, at age eleven years, the patient was referred to the Hearing and Speech Clinic by his school for a complete audiological evaluation. His teacher described the patient as "restless, distractible and appearing to have some difficulty in hearing." He was living with his stepmother who reported that the boy had a history of truancy and that he was doing very poorly in school. She was of the opinion that "he can hear if he wants to."

An otologic examination was entriely within normal limits. On initial audiological evaluation the patient responded consistently to pure tones presented by air conduction at levels between 50-70 db. in each ear. However, he was able to respond to soft conversational speech without difficulty even with earphones in place and visual cues eliminated.

On calibrated speech audiometric testing the patient refused to repeat any spondee words even at levels of 90-100 db. re: audiometric zero. He claimed he did not understand the words or could not hear them. However, he responded to such questions as "Do your hear me now?" or "How do you feel?" at levels between 30-40 db. He was scheduled for a PGSR test.

A detailed explanation of the PGSR test and the instrumentation involved was made to the patient. It was explained that on this test he would not have to tell the examiner when he heard the sounds nor respond in any way but that "the machine will do it all for you electrically."

The patient reluctantly allowed the examiner to affix the electrodes. Several times during the test he removed them by vigorously shaking his hands but allowed them to be re-attached. He was readily conditioned and evidenced reliable PGSR responses to all sounds presented down to a level of 20 db. at all frequencies in the 250-4000 cps range in each ear. He was then asked to indicate when he heard the sounds. He consistently responded by saying "no" each time the tone was presented down to near normal levels.

Results of psychological testing indicated that the patient was functioning on the dull normal to low average level of intelligence. Personality tests revealed a boy who was fearful and suspicious of an environment which he perceived as being threatening to him. Basic hostility and oppositional trends were present and took the form of psychosomatic disorders and neurotic symptoms. Potentials for ungoverned emotional displays were present. He tended to evade highly disturbing situations. There was much ambivalence towards others. On the one hand, he attempted to receive as much love and attention as possible while on the other, he feared establishing relationships with other people.

It was recommended that the boy be given adequate opportunities for socializing with others through appropriate agencies in his community. Supportive psychotherapy was provided. The cooperation of school personnel was enlisted in providing constructive channels of expression. There has been no complaint of hearing or other difficulties in the past two years and the nonorganic hearing problem appears to be, at least to this time, satisfactorily resolved.

REFERENCES

(1) Lynn, G. and Carhart, R.: Influence of attack and release in compression amplification on understanding of speech by hypoacusics. *J. Speech and Hearing Disorders, 28*:124, (May) 1963.

Chapter VI

SCREENING THE HEARING OF YOUNG CHILDREN

THE PROCEDURES which have been considered in previous chapters are designed for use by specially trained personnel for hearing evaluation of children with known or suspected hearing losses. Such procedures constitute the testing aspect of the audiological evaluation which, as previously mentioned, represents one important segment of the total evaluation. The complete evaluation also routinely includes general and specialized medical examinations, a speech and language evaluation, a psychological evaluation and a psycho-social survey. It is the authors' opinion that the comprehensive diagnostic evaluation which these children require is best performed in a properly equipped and staffed institution where the personnel are able to coordinate their efforts effectively and to work toward the optimum rehabilitation of the child. A patient-oriented group of specialists which directs its attention toward the development of improved techniques for rehabilitating the speech and hearing handicapped child as well as the efficient and humane application of existing techniques toward this goal represents the "team approach" at its best. Errors in diagnosis will, of course, occur even under the best conditions since the problems with which we deal are complex and the limits of existing knowledge disturbingly great. But in a well coordinated "team approach" in which each child is scheduled for periodic re-evaluation and is followed into maturity by all members of the staff, we become aware of our errors, both of commission and omission, and fewer should occur with the passage of time and the accummulation of greater knowledge and understanding of the problems we face.

It is true that even after the most complete evaluation possible with existing techniques, as performed in the best organized institutions, many of our conclusions must still be stated as impressions, rather than as definitive diagnoses. These impressions should be subject to substantiation or rejection by further study of the child including observation of his response to multiple rehabilitative approaches. But the child evaluated in this type of professional environment gets the best of what we are presently able to give him. No known stone is left unturned. And in this situation we are less likely to administer inappropriate treatment, e.g., speech reading for the child with impacted cerumen or a hearing aid for a psychotic child who evidences little response to auditory stimulation.

We are frequently asked by physicians, particularly general practitioners, otolaryngologists and pediatricans whether there is any simple procedure which they can perform in their offices which might tell them whether a particular child requires the comprehensive diagnostic services of the Hearing and Speech Center. They often express the desire for a simple screening tool which can be incorporated into a routine physical examination of their pediatric patients. Such a procedure should be brief and easy to administer and require a minimum of special equipment. It should have but one purpose, namely to identify those children who require detailed, individual assessment in the specialized center.

The purpose of this chapter is to describe and evaluate those techniques, old and new which have been suggested for use in auditory screening and which are potentially applicable to the requirements of the practicing physician. The purpose of an auditory screening test is to divide a population into two groups: one composed of persons whose hearing falls within normal limits; the second consisting of those whose hearing fails to meet this criterion and who require more detailed evaluation. It must be borne in mind that the criteria for "normal limits" will very from test to test.

WHISPERED AND SPOKEN VOICE TESTS

Among the oldest screening tests are the whispered and spoken voice tests, the latter sometimes referred to as the conversational voice test. We believe that these procedures are "time *dis*honored tests" since the weight of theoretical and clinical evidence through the years has clearly demonstrated their total inadequacy for the purposes for which they have been proposed and used. In the face of this evidence, we are surprised and dismayed by the continued use of these "tests" in physicians' offices, military induction centers and other places where audiometric equipment is either not available or is used only for "follow up" testing.

A procedure for performing these tests appears, among other places, in a manual prepared for medical examiners working for the Veterans Administration. (1)

> "The examiner stands at twenty feet and makes every effort to assume and maintain an ordinary conversational voice at all times. He should be particularly careful not to lower the voice as he approaches the individual being tested. Words such as baseball, firefly, blackboard, doorstep, inkwell, mouse-trap and hardware should be repeated at 20, 15, 10, 5, 2 and 1 feet until a response is elicited. It is well to repeat the procedure several times to arrive at the most accurate threshold possible. The number of feet at which a response is elicited will be the numerator over 20 which is considered to be the denominator, e.g., 5/20. In other words, the veteran has hearing approximately 5/20th of normal."

It will be seen that the Veterans Administration subsequently recognized the limitations inherent in this test (v.i.).

The whispered and spoken voice tests represent an attempt to apply the principle of the Snellen Test of Visual Acuity to the testing of hearing. Glorig (2) believes that the only reason for the use of the denominator twenty is that at the time when ophthalmology and otolaryngology were frequently associated with each other, it was convenient for a hearing test to be done in the same manner as an eye test. Several obvious advantages have been claimed for this form of testing which include the following:

1.   Simplicity of Administration

Personnel with little or no background in audiometry may be taught to administer these tests in a short period of time.

2. Lack of Expense

No special equipment is required and large numbers of persons may be screened in a short period of time.

3. Use of Functional Stimuli

The range of frequencies most important for understanding speech extends from about 400 to 3000 cps and conversational speech tests provide information on the subject's hearing in this range.

These advantages are more than outweighed, however, by the serious limitations of these tests. These include the following:

1. Lack of control of the sound source. Sound intensity varies inversely with the square of the distance. In actual practice, therefore, this means that changes in the distance between the examiner and the subject greater than eight feet produce relatively small changes in intensity, while slight changes at distances less than eight feet will produce considerable alterations in intensity. (3)

2. Variations in speech levels of examiners. There are considerable differences in the conversational voice levels of different testers and in the same tester from time to time. Proper monitoring of spoken voice intensity requires, at least, a sound level meter usually not available to examiners using conversational voice tests. The reflex of raising the voice with distance is an important source of error in non-monitored speech tests.

3. Variations in articulation and voice quality. In addition to variations in overall voice intensity level, examiners differ in the clarity of their articulation, rate of speech production, dialectical characteristics and frequency spectra of the fundamental and overtone structure of their voices. These and other related factors introduce significant variables into the test situation.

4. Lack of standardization of material. Some examiners use a series of spondee words for these tests; others employ a series of digits. There is no uniformly accepted list of material which has been properly standardized on groups of normal hearing persons.

5. Lack of properly sound isolated test areas. These tests are often administered in rooms with excessively high noise levels and hard surfaces which reflect sound waves. In tests involving live voice presentation of material, the ambient noise level assumes special significance since the examiner, if he has normal hearing, will reflexly raise the intensity of his voice above the level of background noise. This mechanism is the basis of the Lombard Voice Reflex Test, one of the procedures utilized in the detection of nonorganic hearing losses.

6. Failure to test a sufficiently wide frequency range. The most important phonetic elements in spondaic words are the vowels which have most of their acoustic energy in the range below 1000 cps. This is also largely true of digits which represent an even easier type of test material for the patient because the number of possible choices is reduced. Persons with sensorineural hearing losses affecting frequencies above 1000 cps are usually able to pass these tests with little difficulty. Hearing losses in children frequently affect the high frequency portion of the range (3000-8000 cps) before the critical "speech frequencies" are affected. Such hearing problems frequently escape detection until testing is performed with wide range discrete frequency stimuli.

7. Failure to isolate ears adequately. The procedure of having the patient cover one ear with the hand or having him press on the tragus of the untested ear does not prevent this ear from participating in the test. The conversational voice level of some examiners is readily audible even with the patient's fingers pressing both tragi.

The United States Armed Forces and the Veterans Administration have shown increased recognition of the limitations inherent in whispered and spoken voice tests. The Veterans Administration began in 1952 to use pure tone and speech audiometry for rating purposes. (4) Prior to that time, distance tests had been used not only to determine whether a veteran's hearing loss was service connected but also to specify his disability rating.

The widespread use of calibrated hearing tests by the Armed Forces is reflected in a 1956 Air Force regulation (5) which states that the medical service will perform audiometric examinations to

1. establish initial hearing thresholds for all individuals entering air force service; 2. establish the reference audiogram for individuals exposed to noise; 3. secure follow-up information and data on threshold shifts for use in disposing of personnel.

The scale of hearing prepared by the Committee on Hearing of the National Research Council in 1949 for possible incorporation in a set of physical standards appropriate to the peace-time needs of the Army and the Navy, and to partial or total mobilization described degrees of hearing loss in terms of decibels rather than in feet. Pure tone air conduction audiometry was recommended for classification purposes. (6)

Reports on the serious limitations of whispered and spoken voice tests have appeared in the literature for many years. Glorig (7) compared the results of 173 conversational speech tests with pure tone and calibrated speech audiometry on the same group of patients and found that "the inconsistency was remarkable." Monitored speech tests (using a microphone, amplifier and output meter to assure a fairly constant output) varied one to five feet lower than the unmonitored test. He concluded that the spoken voice test has inherent faults which make it impossible to arrive at even approximate hearing thresholds. According to all the laws of acoustics, he considers the test in no way practical or even admissible.

Fowler, Jr. (8) focused specific attention on the voice reflex as a source of inaccuracy in conversational speech tests. The voice reflex refers to the raising of the examiner's voice as he moves away from the subject and to its lowering as the subject is approached. The conversational and whispered voice levels of a series of trained examiners was checked with a sound level meter at distances of five and fifteen feet. Fowler found that the reflex of raising the voice with distance was so great that with the exception of three of the twelve examiners, there was no change in the intensity of the whisper and the spoken word reaching the sound level meter and the patient at fifteen feet and five feet in a sound treated room. Often the intensity of the spoken voice reaching the meter and the patient was greater at fifteen than at five feet. Hoople, (9) Fowler, Sr., (10) Work, (11) Knudsen and Jones (12) and Canfield (13) are quoted by Glorig as among those who have talked and written of the shortcomings of conversational speech tests for years.

While one of us (MHM) was stationed at a Class II Army hospital in 1954, pure tone audiometry was performed on 1311 servicemen who had previously passed a whispered and spoken voice test as administered by experienced army personnel. Apart from the large number of persons with mild losses of hearing and unilateral losses which were not picked up, three bilateral losses were detected which averaged more than 30 db. for the three central frequencies in the better ear. In other words, it was possible for an individual with a hearing loss of sufficient magnitude to constitute a social and vocational handicap to pass a whispered and spoken voice test as administered by experienced personnel.

TUNING FORK TESTS

Tuning forks, in the hands of an experienced and knowledgeable examiner can yield valuable diagnostic data. They are helpful in the differentiation of conductive and sensorineural hearing losses and are employed by many otolaryngologists as part of their clinical evaluation of the hard of hearing patient. It is difficult to use tuning forks to determine auditory thresholds because (1) the so-called "standard blow" used to activate the tuning fork differs from examiner to examiner; (2) there is no zero reference point readily available as the standard for normal hearing at the frequency investigated; (3) an especially quiet area with non-reflecting walls is required since no attenuation of ambient noise is provided by rubber earphone cushions as in audiometric testing; and (4) the Barany noise apparatus often used as a masking stimulus with tuning fork tests produces a noise of 140 db. (sound pressure level) in the external auditory canal and this frequently overmasks the test stimulus. The use of tuning forks is particularly limited with children since they often respond affirmatively regardless of whether or not the tone is heard. The classical tuning fork tests such as the Weber, Rinne and Gellé continue to yield valuable qualitative data on the nature of the hearing loss and their intelligent use in appropriate cases should not be discouraged.

WATCH TICK AND COIN CLICK TESTS

Such tests as the watch tick and coin click tests for auditory screening can only be viewed with amusement by present day standards. The watch tick test was used in the past by some examiners to determine whether a patient's hearing fell within normal limits. The examiner supposedly knew at what distance from the ear a person with normal hearing could detect the watch tick. The distance required for a person with a suspected hearing loss was compared with this standard in an effort to determine whether a hearing loss was present. The coin click test was employed in an effort to determine whether a high frequency hearing loss was present. A coin, usually a half dollar was dropped on a metal surface and the patient asked to describe what was heard. If he heard a "ping," he was assumed to have intact hearing in the high frequency portion of the range. If he heard only a dull thud, some impairment in this range was assumed.

Both of these tests sample primarily the high frequencies and provide information only about the patient's hearing in a limited portion of the range. The greatest amount of acoustic energy in such sounds occurs primarily above the range critical for speech reception. To derive any degree of useful information from these tests requires at least a spectral analysis of the sounds employed to indicate the distribution of acoustic energy as a function of frequency. Needless to say, few examiners who employed such methods of testing had such data available to them. We hope we are justified in using the past tense in our description of the use of these tests but suspect from our observations that we are not completely correct in doing so.

GROUP SCREENING TESTS

A variety of procedures have been developed to screen the hearing of large numbers of persons in a short period of time. The Western Electric 4A and 4C attenuated or Fading Numbers test is still employed in a number of public school systems for periodic auditory screening. The input for this test is a phonograph turntable whose output can be fed to forty earphones simultaneously. The test stimulus is a series of two digit numbers spoken by a female telephone operator. Digits are similar to spondee words in that the critical phonetic elements in both are the low frequency vowels. As previously mentioned, tests which employ spondees or numbers as the test stimulus fail to detect losses affecting the high frequency portion of the range where most of the "intelligence" of the language is concentrated. There are other serious limitations in this form of testing which explain the high incidence of false positives and false negatives which occur when it is employed in a program of hearing conservation. These limitations will not be considered because the fading numbers test is a group test and is not designed for use by the physician in the individual screening of a child. Physicians who serve as consultants for hearing conservation programs in the public school system should become familiar with some of the literature dealing with test procedures for use in public school auditory screening. A few of these references are included in the bibliography. (14, 15, 16, 17, 18)

Pure tone audiometry has been adapted in a number of ways for use as a group test. A variety of types of instrumentation and test procedures have been suggested. (19, 20, 21, 22, 23, 24, 25) Group pure tone screening tests permit the evaluation of more than one person at a time while preserving many of the advantages of the individual pure tone test. It is generally agreed that an individual pure tone test is the best method available for detecting hearing loss but that its use is limited in screening large populations because of the time involved in its administration. Although group pure tone screening is not as effective as the individual pure tone test in detecting children with hearing loss, certain of the proposed forms of group testing approach the effectiveness of the individual test and should be given serious consideration in the organization of a public school hearing testing program.

INDIVIDUAL PURE TONE SCREENING

Many children three years of age and over can be tested without difficulty with a pure tone audiometer. These are children with suspected hearing loss who do not have other problems of the type previously discussed. An increasing number of general practitioners, pediatricians and otolaryngologists are including a pure tone screening test as part of their regular physical examination. Such testing is also performed after the child has had an upper respiratory infection, any disease with hyperpyrexia, or after use of a drug with known or suspected ototoxicity. The audiometer need not be an elaborate one and, for screening purposes, may be limited to air conduction at five frequencies (500, 1000, 2000, 4000, and 8000 cps). It may be either battery operated or utilize standard house current. Some units can operate on either type of current. An increasing number of audiometers have become available which utilize a transistorized circuit and are readily portable. The use of a transistorized circuit eliminates the need for a preliminary warm up period. Such units are not otherwise necessarily superior to vacuum tube audiometers.

A suggested procedure for administering an individual pure tone screening test in the physician's office is the following:

1. The external auditory canals should be cleared of any obstructive material.

2. Instruct the child to raise his hand as soon as he hears each of a series of tones which will be presented first to his right, then to his left ear keeping his hand raised as long as the sound is on and lowering it when the sound can no longer be heard. The type of response involved should be demonstrated to the child.

3. Set the attenuator (hearing loss) control to a point where the 1000 cps tone is clearly audible. (30-35 db. re: normal threshold for children whose hearing is grossly normal.) Get the child familiar with the sound stimulus before checking hearing at a particular frequency. Pure tones represent an unfamiliar type of stimulus for most persons, young or old, because they seldom occur in everyday life. The child being tested should, therefore, have the sound presented to him first at an easily audible level before any testing is performed. The attenuator is then set to a level within normal limits. This is usually at 15 db. re: normal threshold but may be lowered to 10 db. in sufficiently quiet areas. If the tones to be tested are not audible to the examiner at the 15 db. level, and if the examiner's hearing is normal, a different location should be used for the screening.

4. With earphones placed one over each ear, start the test at

1000 cps in the right ear. Make certain that the receiver of the earphone is in satisfactory approximation with the external canal. Testing is started at 1000 cps because studies of the stability of the auditory threshold have shown that the highest test-retest consistency is obtained at this frequency. Avoid a rhythmic pattern of tone presentation. Vary the duration of exposure to the tone as well as the interval between presentations. If the child responds satisfactorily to the 1000 cps tone at the predetermined intensity level, test 2000, 4000, 8000 and 500 cps in that order. Testing below 500 cps is not recommended under most conditions because typical office noise, having most of its energy in the lower frequencies will mask 250 and 125 cps quite effectively. The inclusion of these lower frequencies will result in an excessive number of false positives. Such children are later found to have normal hearing when tested under more favorable noise conditions. Keep the tone in the normally off position, thus exposing the child to the tone for the shortest possible time and reducing adaptation and fatigue effects. Most modern audiometers have a tone interrupter switch which enables the tester to keep the sound either normally on or normally off. For pure tone screening and threshold testing, the tone should be in the normally off position. The noise of the frequency dial as the examiner switches from one frequency to another should be kept to a minimum. This should also apply to all other extraneous sounds.

A child who is unable to hear one or more of the five frequencies presented to him should be considered to have failed the screening test and arrangements should be made for a pure tone threshold air and bone conduction test. Many persons of all ages are found to have losses at 4000 cps of varying degrees of severity due to a variety of causes. If the hearing loss affects only this frequency and is of the sensorineural type, it is generally not significant unless the individual is actively exposed to a high intensity noise environment for prolonged periods of time. In children, high frequency losses may be of the *conductive* type and are often related to hypertrophied lymphoid tissue in the nasopharynx. It will not be possible to determine the type of hearing loss present at this or any other frequency by air conduction testing alone. Unless the physician also includes bone conduction testing which requires even quieter conditions than air conduction tests, arrangements should be made for follow up testing of those children who fail to respond at the screening level to *any* of the frequencies tested.

Among the advantages of the individually administered pure tone screening test are the following:

1. Broad frequency spectrum is tested. The use of pure tone audiometers makes it possible to pick up losses at an early stage before they have affected the child's ability to respond to speech. At this stage, the possibilities of medical and/or surgical correction or stabilization are generally excellent in the case of conductive losses in children. Losses of hearing above 1000 cps, often undetected by tests using speech as the stimulus, are readily picked up by pure tone audiometry.

2. Adequate control of frequency and intensity of test stimuli. Acceptable pure tone audiometers must meet the specifications established by the Council on Physical Medicine and Rehabilitation of the American Medical Association and the American Standards Association. The many variables which affect the validity of whispered and spoken voice testing are eliminated when a properly calibrated pure tone audiometer is used. A listing of audiometers which have met the standards of a Subcommittee of the Committee on Conservation of Hearing of the American Academy of Ophthalmology and Otolaryngology is published regularly in the Transactions of the American Academy of Ophthalmology and Otolaryngology.

3. Ease of administration. Persons with limited or no previous experience in administering hearing tests can be quickly trained to administer pure tone screening tests. It takes only a few seconds longer to perform this type of test than a conversational voice test. We have estimated the average time taken by personnel to perform a spoken voice test to be forty-eight seconds. It is possible to perform a five frequency auditory screening test on an adult in about sixty seconds. With children, more time is required for both tests. The important advantages of pure tone screening surely warrant the small additional expenditure of time.

Persons who continue to utilize whispered and spoken voice tests sometimes defend this practice by stating that they use these tests *for screening only*. They acknowledge all the advantages of pure tone testing and arrange for such tests on all persons who fail the spoken voice screening test. The fallacy of this philosophy is that a program of hearing conservation stands or falls according to its effectiveness in detecting the largest possible number of children with significant hearing impairments. If the screening test employed fails to detect some of these children with significant hearing problems, the quality of the follow-up testing is meaningless to them. The ideal first echelon test should pick up *all* children requiring further investigation. Pure tone testing should, therefore, be employed not only as part of the follow-up diagnostic tests but for initial screening as well.

SINGLE AND DOUBLE FREQUENCY AUDITORY SCREENING

"A new concept in auditory screening" was described several years ago by Glorig and House (26) for use in screening the hearing of large populations. In this method of screening, only 4000 cps or a combination of 2000 and 4000 cps are used. Proponents of this method have presented audiometric evidence on three large population groups which they believe makes it possible to predict that losses at any standard test frequency will not be greater than that which occurs at 4000 cps. Both a one- and two-frequency version of the instrument, known as the Oto-Chek are commercially available. Among the advantages claimed for this method are the following: (1) Ordinary quiet rooms (offices, First Aid rooms, etc.) may be used for testing since typical room noise will not mask the high frequencies used in this test. (2) The test requires only a few seconds to complete, saving time and preventing fatigue. (3) The instrument is inexpensive, lightweight and durable.

Miller and Bella (27) suggested that in order to evaluate properly the efficiency of this method of screening, it is necessary to compute the percentage of children who *fail*—not who pass—with each method of screening. It is the group of children *with* hearing loss which must concern us in an adequate program of hearing conservation, not the larger group with normal hearing. When the Glorig-

House data are thus analyzed, we find that of the 1500 children tested, eighty-four children failed the single frequency test while 101 children failed with the five frequency sweep-check. This means that the five frequency sweep-check picked up seventeen more children with hearing loss than did the single frequency test. Seventeen children represents almost 17 per cent of the total number of children with hearing loss. A proposed screening method which misses this percentage of children should be carefully evaluated before it is adopted.

In the same article an analysis of 3630 tests performed in the Greenwich school system in a one year period was reported. Particular attention was paid to the number of these children with significant losses of hearing who would not have been detected if testing had been limited to the one or two frequencies suggested by Glorig and House. If 4000 cps only had been used, only 39 per cent of the losses would have been picked up. Had the 2 frequency test been used, an additional 7.2 per cent of the losses would have been detected. It was further found that the audiometric frequency showing the greatest hearing loss was not 4000 cps in a large portion of the losses found.

A number of reports have appeared since the introduction of single and double frequency screen testing, some supporting this approach (28-30) and others rejecting it. (31-34) Several studies support the concept of two-frequency testing provided that frequencies other than those suggested by Glorig and House are used. (35, 36) Combinations of 500 and 4000 cps or 1000 and 4000 cps were found to be more effective in picking up larger numbers of children with significant losses of hearing than 2000 and 4000 cps. Differences of opinion are based partly on the objectives of the auditory screening program and the effectiveness of the method with which the new approach is compared. Those who are concerned with identifying children with all degrees of hearing loss, including those with medically significant impairments, are generally dissatisfied with single and double frequency screening.

An adequate program of hearing conservation must facilitate the detection of the largest possible number of children with hearing losses of any significant degree. The conditions under which such testing is performed imposes limits on the degree of hearing loss which can be detected. While the Glorig-House approach may be superior to some forms of auditory screening, it falls far short, in our judgment, of the results obtainable by individual pure tone tests. We would, therefore, discourage its use by the physician and encourage him to use the full five-frequency test whenever possible.

In the present chapter, we have considered methods of auditory screening for the cooperative child who presents no problems other than possible peripheral hearing loss. A number of the children who reach the physician are not testable by rapid pure tone screening regardless of their age and require the comprehensive services of the Hearing and Speech Center. The parents of such children usually report lack of or inconsistent response to auditory stimuli, or retarded or absent speech development. These reports should be treated with respect by the physician and not shrugged off by a casual statement that the child will "outgrow" the problem. If the physician feels there *may* be a basis for the parents' concern, arrangements should be made for appropriate evaluation of the problem. If the parent is prone to exaggeration of her observations and has established inordinately high standards for her children in other areas, the complaint must be viewed by the physician with these considerations in mind. It is the physician, particularly one who has known the family for many years, who is in the best position to evaluate the parents' report. In general, we would prefer that the physician err on the side of making too many rather than too few referrals of children with suspected hearing and speech disorders.

We look forward to the day when hearing evaluation of children will be as frequently requested as are blood counts, urinalyses, x-ray studies and other laboratory tests whenever and wherever the physician suspects that a problem may exist.

REFERENCES

(1) U.S. Veterans Administration: *Manual for Medical Examiners of the Veterans Administration.* Rev. June 1951, U.S. Govt. Print. Off., Washington, D. C., 1951, p. 25.

(2) Glorig, A.: Hearing evaluation by low conversational voice tests. *Ann. Otol. Rhin. and Laryng.,* 58:394, (June) 1949.

(3) Glorig, A.: Problems in hearing. *U.S. Armed Forces M.J., 1*:590, (May) 1950.

(4) U.S. Veterans Administration, Dept. of Medicine and Surgery, Information bulletin: *Audiology.* I B 10-115, (March 7) 1960, p. 5.

(5) U.S. Air Force Regulation 160-3, par. 13: "Monitoring Audiometry," Oct. 29, 1956.

(6) Davis, H. and Silverman, S. R., eds.: *Hearing and Deafness.* Rev. ed., Holt, Rinehart and Winston, New York, 1960, pp. 242-243.

(7) Glorig, A.: Hearing evaluation by low conversational voice tests. *op. cit.*

(8) Fowler, E. P., Jr.: Discovery and evaluation of otic cripples. *Arch. Otolaryng., 45*:550, (May) 1947.

(9) Hoople, G. D., Wolfe, W. C. and Bregande, S. C.: Unrecognized battle noise trauma. *Laryngoscope, 57*:125, (Feb.) 1947.

(10) Fowler, E. P.: The percentage of capacity to hear speech and related disabilities. *Laryngoscope, 57*:103, (Feb.) 1947.

(11) Work, W. P.: Aural rehabilitation: army experience. *Laryngoscope, 57*:423, (July) 1947.

(12) Knudsen, V. O. and Jones, I. H.: Basic principles underlying tests of hearing. *Laryngoscope, 45*:1, (Jan.) 1935.

(13) Canfield, N.: Personal communication to Dr. A. Glorig.

(14) Newhart, H. and Reger, S. N., eds.: *Manual for a School Hearing Conservation Program.* Rev. by Kinney, C. E., et al., in *Trans. Amer. Acad. Ophthal. Otolaryng.,* Suppl., 1951.

(15) Dahl, L. A.: *Public School Audiometry: Principles and Methods.* Interstate, Danville, Ill., 1949.

(16) Newhart, H.: The conservation of hearing. *Tr. Amer. Otol. Soc., 30*:16, 1940.

(17) West, R., Becker, V. A. and Rohr, J. A.: Program for Hearing Conservation. Madison, Wis., Bureau for Handicapped Children, Dept. of Public Instruction, 1943.

(18) Newby, H. A.: *Audiology: Principles and Practice.* Appleton-Century-Crofts, New York, 1958, chap. VIII.

(19) Allison, R. E.: A new pure tone group audiometer test. *J. Acous. Soc. Amer., 22*:675, 1950. (Abstract)

(20) Johnston, P. W.: The Massachusetts hearing test. *J. Acous. Soc. Amer., 20*:697, 1948.

(21) Reger, S. N. and Newby, H. A.: A group pure tone hearing test. *J. Speech Disorders, 12*:61, (Mar.) 1947.

(22) A group automatic audiometer in a hearing conservation program. USN MRL Memorandum Report No. 58-3, March 24, 1958.

(23) Final report automatic group audiometer. Maico Report R-273, MA-4, Nov. 21, 1958.

(24) Glorig, A. and Wilke, R. R.: A new automatic screening audiometer. *J. Acous. Soc. Amer., 24*:450, 1952.

(25) Webster, J. C. and Thompson, P. O.: Recorded group audiometer test comparisons at the 1956 Southern California Exposition. *J. Acous. Soc. Amer., 29*:895, 1957.

(26) Glorig, A. and House, H. P.: A new concept in auditory screening. *A.M.A. Arch. Otolaryng., 66*:228, (Aug.) 1957.

(27) Miller, M. H. and Bella, J. L.: Limitations of selected frequency audiometry in the public schools. *J. Speech and Hearing Disorders, 24*:402, (Nov.) 1959.

(28) Ventry, I. M. and Newby, H. A.: Validity of the one-frequency screening principle for public school children. *J. Speech and Hearing Res., 2*:147, 1959.

(29) Hanley, C. N. and Gaddie, B. G.: The use of single frequency audiometry in the screening of school children. *J. Speech and Hearing Disorders, 27*:258, (Aug.) 1962.

(30) Sataloff, J. and Menduke, H.: Single- and double-frequency screening in school children. *A.M.A. Arch. Otolaryng., 70*:624, (Nov.) 1959.

(31) Lightfoot, C., Buckingham, R. A. and Kelly, M. N.: A check on oto-chek. *A.M.A. Arch Otolaryng., 70*:103, (July) 1959.

(32) Maxwell, W. R. and Davidson, G. D.: Limited-frequency screening and ear pathology. *J. Speech and Hearing Disorders, 26*:122, (May) 1961.

(33) Siegenthaler, B. M. and Sommers, R. K.: Abbreviated sweep-check procedures for school hearing testing. *J. Speech and Hearing Disorders, 24*:249, (Aug.) 1959.

(34) Stevens, D. A. and Davidson, G. D.: Screening tests of hearing. *J. Speech and Hearing Disorders, 24*:258, (Aug.) 1959.

(35) Farrant, R. H.: The audiometric testing of children in schools and kindergartens. *J. Aud. Res., 1*:1, 1960.

(36) Lawrence, C. L. and Rubin, W.: The efficiency of limited frequency audiometric screening in a school hearing conservation program, presented to 1958 convention of Amer. Speech and Hearing Assoc., New York.

APPENDIX

THE IMPETUS FOR establishing new facilities for hearing evaluation and rehabilitation frequently comes from the physician, usually the otolaryngologist or the pediatrician. He must be familiar with the personnel required for the operation of such a facility as well as with the instrumentation required to perform the various services which should be offered.

The Bureau for Handicapped Children of the New York City Department of Health has established a set of recommended standards for institutions who wish to have their Hearing and Speech services approved under their Hearing Conservation Program. The authors wish to express their appreciation to Miss Margaret Losty, Acting Director of the Bureau and her colleagues for permission to reprint the current version of the Recommended Standards. It is hoped that these standards will be of assistance to physicians and others who are called upon to assist in the development of new facilities for auditory evaluation and rehabilitation.

RECOMMENDED STANDARDS FOR HEARING CENTERS
Bureau for Handicapped Children
New York City Department of Health
Revised 1961

INTRODUCTION

Leaders in the field concerned with the care and rehabilitation of patients with defective hearing have long recognized that for total rehabilitation, many skills are necessary. These include the pediatrician (or internist for adults), otologist, audiologist, the speech and hearing therapist, clinical psychologist, social worker, nurse, vocational counselor, psychiatrist and clerical and technical staff. In considering total care and rehabilitation of patients the medical aspects are important, but at times the major problems to be considered may be psychological, educational, social or vocational. As in any program or service where many professional people are needed, the most effective method for the care and rehabilitation of patients with hearing problems is through the "team approach," the method whereby the various professional personnel work closely together and integrate their skills for the maximum benefit of the patient. It is important to the concept of comprehensive care that there be a close cooperative team effort among all members of the team throughout the patient's need for care.

Because of the nature of the problems of a person with defective hearing, total needs are not now being met in the community. Only limited services have been available in the past to offer a child the opportunity to have complete evaluation of his total hearing problem, diagnosis, comprehensive treatment and rehabilitation.

The standards described in this material were first established in June 1953 with the assistance of a Technical Advisory Committee. This revised edition has again been prepared with the assistance of the Technical Advisory Committee and has been based on experience gained over a seven year period in the New York City Community Hearing Program.

TECHNICAL ADVISORY GROUP
ON HEARING AND SPEECH PROGRAM
1953

Dr. John F. Daly, Chairman

Dr. Morris S. Bender
Dr. Reuel A. Benson
Dr. Jon Eisenson
Dr. Edmund P. Fowler, Jr.
Dr. Joseph G. Gilbert
Dr. Joseph Golomb
Dr. William G. Hardy
Dr. Morris F. Heller
Dr. Arthur J. Herzig
Dr. Gervais Ward McAuliffe

Dr. George W. McCormick
Mr. Donald M. Markle
Miss Marion Martin
Dr. Clarence D. O'Connor
Dr. Herbert H. Pomerance
Dr. Henry Rascoff
Mrs. Eleanor C. Ronnei
Dr. Lawrence B. Slobody
Miss Theodate H. Soule
Dr. Robert West

EXTENT OF THE PROBLEM

There are no accurate statistics on the number of acoustically handicapped persons in the United States. Estimates of the number of persons who have a hearing loss (ranging from a slight loss to almost total deafness) range from 7 million to 14 million, while an estimated 800,000 persons wear hearing aids as compared with an estimated 1,600,000 who need them. Estimates of the number of children with hearing impairment range from 2 to 12 per cent of the population up to a figure of 3 million. The Vocational Rehabilitation Administration has estimated that there are at least 33,000 deaf civilians and 206,000 who are hard-of-hearing who are eligible for services from state vocational rehabilitation agencies. In New York City, it is estimated that 30,000 to 40,000 children of school age have a hearing loss requiring a careful evaluation. The number of pre-school children and adults so affected is unknown. The large number of patients requiring these services in the community and the cost of developing and operating such services have made this a responsibility of the community. This has been realized by many communities that are now actively engaged in developing hearing conservation programs.

I. Purpose and Functions of the Hearing Center

    A. To provide complete services for the diagnosis, treatment and rehabilitation of children and adults who have or are suspected of having a hearing impairment.

    B. To care for not only patients usually known to the hospital but also patients referred by practicing physicians, community agencies, school health and child health services, and industry.

    C. To provide interpretation and guidance to the patient and his family and assist the patient and his family in making the necessary plans for the patient's total, maximum rehabilitation.

    D. To be a training center for professional personnel of all types, both at the undergraduate and postgraduate levels.

    E. To perform research.

II. Accreditations

    To provide maximum diagnostic, evaluation, treatment and rehabilitation facilities, hearing centers should be within the environs or closely affiliated with a general hospital. The hospital should have the following accreditation:

A. Approval by the Joint Commission on Accreditation of Hospitals.

B. Approval by the Council on Medical Education and Hospitals of the American Medical Association for Residency training in pediatrics.

C. Approval by the Council on Medical Education and Hospitals of the American Medical Association for residency training in otolaryngology.

III. Services Required

The rehabilitation objective can best be attained through the team approach of all of the professional disciplines involved in the care of children and adults with suspected or established hearing problems. It is important to the concept of comprehensive care of children and youth that there be a close, cooperative team effort among all members of the team. Continuous care should be provided from the time of earliest recognition until maximum rehabilitation is achieved. The following basic services are essential to provide care in depth and should be available in proportion to the needs of the patients under care: pediatrics, otolaryngology, audiology, psychology, speech therapy and social service. Consultation service from the fields of neurology, psychiatry, orthopedic surgery, ophthalmology and other medical specialties should be readily available when indicated.

IV. Personnel

A. *Medical Direction and Supervision*

Medical direction of the center's activities is essential because the investigation and recommendations are based upon medical findings. It is probably not practical to have a full-time medical director. In order to maintain a high quality of service and coordination, a full-time coordinator or supervisor of the center is necessary. This responsibility can best be assumed by the audiologist with

Advanced Certification in Hearing or its equivalent from the American Speech and Hearing Association. Medical supervision by qualified otolaryngologists and pediatricans is necessary for the initial evaluation of the patient and for continuing medical treatment and rehabilitation. Ideally, at least one otolaryngologist and one pediatrician should be assigned to the center staff to participate in direct patient care, to function as a member of the center team, and to attend the center's staff conferences. In addition to these two essential medical services, consultation should be readily available from all of the related medical fields such as neurology, psychiatry, radiology, plastic surgery, orthopedic surgery, and orthodontia. In addition, it is highly desirable that members of the house staff from the otolaryngological and pediatric services be rotated through the center in order that they may receive training in the care of acoustically handicapped patients. This same principle might also be applied to other groups such as nurses, social workers, physical therapists and psychologists.

B. *Paramedical Professional Staff*

A battery of professional skills is required for the complete evaluation, treatment and rehabilitation of patients with hearing impairment. Personnel with such skills include those trained in the fields of audiology, speech therapy, hearing therapy, psychology, medical social work, nursing and electronics. Each of the professional personnel should meet the qualifications established for the particular discipline. Equally important is the functioning of each professional person in such a way that the group functions as a team, so that the total needs of the patient will be considered and met.

C. *Clerical Staff*

Adequate clerical workers are essential to the proper functioning of the center if professional time is to be used for patient care only.

V. Program

A. Each person seen in the center should have the following basic examinations:
   1. A general medical or pediatric examination.
   2. An examination of the ears, nose and throat by an otologist.
   3. Audiological evaluation including pure tone air and bone conduction testing and a speech audiometric evaluation.

   Hearing aid evaluation, speech and language, social service, psychological, medical consultations and other examinations are then scheduled according to the needs of the patient as indicated by the results of the three basic examinations.

B. An annual re-evaluation of each person under the program will consist of the following:
   1. Examination of the ears, nose and throat.
   2. Repeat pure tone and speech audiometric examination.
   3. Repeat hearing aid evaluation of present performance with amplification and need, if any, for change in hearing aid fitting.
   4. An evaluation by the psychologist or social worker of the patient's adjustment to the problem, including acceptance of amplification, personal and social problems associated with the hearing loss, etc.

C. Staff conferences should be held routinely, preferably weekly, to review all new and old patients at periodic intervals and to review problems in the operation of the center. These conferences should include active participation by all professional staff.

D. Personality and developmental evaluation of every child should be made by the pediatrician. Any questionable cases on an individual basis should be referred to the psychologist.

E. Parent counseling should be one of the important functions of the center. A designated member of the team should assume the responsibility for interpretation of the total program and plan to the parents (and child) with assistance from other members of the team when indicated. Each member of the team should be alert to the need for early family counseling and be aware of the responsibilities in this regard.

VI. Follow-up

A. A well planned administrative device should be established in the center for an appointment system and a follow-up of broken appointments.

B. The long term treatment required for adequate rehabilitation of the patient should be supplemented by follow-up assistance in the home and in the school as indicated.

C. Speech training activities within the center should be coordinated with the Public School program to further enrich the child's experience.

D. The community public health nursing agencies should be utilized as much as possible to assist in carrying out the total program.

E. There should be cooperation with public and private schools which offer educational programs for children with communication disorders.

VII. Vocational Guidance

At age fourteen years or as soon thereafter as possible, all children under this program will require assistance in vocational planning. When decisions in this area have been made by the team, the medical social worker should arrange for referral of the patient to the Division of Vocational Rehabilitation of the New York State Department of Education. In centers where a rehabilitation counselor is a member of the team, planning for referral should be made jointly by the medical personnel, social worker and the rehabilitation counselor.

VIII. Physical Setup

A. One of the first principles is the provision of an integrated unit with complete services for the diagnosis, treatment and rehabilitation of patients. Such a unit should be located in a quiet section of the hospital, away from heavy machinery, main plumbing lines and similar distractive noises.

B. The physical setup should include the following:

1. Rooms for the reception area and waiting space.
2. Offices of the director, social worker, and psychologist.
3. Play room for observation of children.
4. Two audiometric testing rooms for routine pure tone audiometric testing that have been adequately treated for sound isolation. The overall noise level on the "flat" scale of a sound level meter should be not more than 45 db. The materials utilized in the construction of the sound treated areas should yield a minimum, overall Noise Reduction Coefficient of 0.95.

   Pure tone air and bone conduction measurements will be performed in these rooms. The ambient noise levels of these rooms should permit air and bone conduction measurements for persons with normal hearing, down to —10 db. at all octave points in the 125-8000 cps range for air conduction and —10 db. at all octave points in the 250-4000 cps range for bone conduction. The minimum inside dimensions of these rooms should be 5′x8′.
5. Two auditory training rooms, including a smaller room for individual training and a larger room for group training.
6. Two speech therapy rooms, including a smaller room for individual therapy and a larger room for group therapy.
7. Medical examination rooms equipped for use by the otological and pediatric staffs.
8. Two sound-treated suites, with each suite having a test room for the patient and a control room for the examiner. The overall noise level on the "flat" scale of a sound level meter should be not more than 45

db. for the control room and 35 db. for the test room. The test room will be a "floating" room in order to achieve these levels. The materials utilized in the construction of the sound treated area should yield a minimum, overall Noise Reduction Coefficient of 0.95. These testing suites are designed for the performance of sound field measurements using monitored microphone voice and recorded inputs. In order to perform satisfactory speech audiometric tests in a sound field at suprathreshold levels for patients with varying degrees of hearing loss, the isolation between the test and control room should permit the introduction of the examiner's voice over a microphone at levels up to 122 db. SPL (100 db. re: audiometric zero). The ambient noise levels of the "floating" test room should permit the determination of Speech Reception Thresholds down to —10 db. re: audiometric zero. Frequency modulated pure tones for sound field testing should be heard in these test rooms down to —10 db. by listeners with normal hearing. The minimum inside dimensions of the test room are 6′x6′ and for the control room 6′x5′.

Air conditioning for the audiometric test rooms is desirable but must be acoustically treated. The overall noise level should not be increased beyond the stated limits by the installation of the air conditioning system. Where air conditioning is not feasible some means of ventilating these rooms without affecting the noise level should be provided. A fan which automatically starts when one or more doors leading to the test room of the two room testing suite are opened is a possible although not ideal solution to the problem of ventilating the "floating" rooms. In this way circulation of air in the rooms is possible between tests. Such an arrangement requires frequent rest periods during the performance of lengthy audiological evaluations particularly in hot, humid weather.

9. Ear Mold Impression Area.
10. Storage space for hearing aids and accessories, stock earmolds, etc.
11. Electronics workshop which may be part of the general instrument repair shop of the hospital.

In order to provide all these facilities, an area of approximately 2,500 square feet is recommended.

IX. Records and Statistics

A. A unit system of records (inpatient and outpatient) should be maintained so that all data (medical, social, psychological, etc.) about the child are available in one unit record folder.

B. Reports should be sent to the school which the child is attending and routinely to any referring physician.

C. Annual statistical data should be kept in regard to:
1. Age of patients
2. Patient load
3. Patient visits and revisits
4. Number of speech therapy sessions or visits
5. Number of audiometric examinations and audiologic workups
6. Number of surgical procedures and types
7. Number of psychological and social evaluations
8. Number of hearing aid evaluations

D. Annual and long term evaluation records should be kept in respect to the number of patients who achieve:
1. Maximum improvement
2. Moderate improvement
3. Slight improvement
4. No improvement

PERSONNEL REQUIREMENTS AND QUALIFICATIONS

The personnel of the Hearing and Speech Center should meet the following basic requirements and qualifications:

1. Pediatrician

The Hearing and Speech Center should have on its staff one

or more pediatricians who are Diplomates of the American Board of Pediatrics. The total number of pediatricians provided will depend on the case load of children and youths served by the center.

2. Otolaryngologist

The otolaryngologist should be a Diplomate of the American Board of Otolaryngology or eligible for certification by such Board. It is desirable that he have special interest and aptitude in hearing problems. The total number of otolaryngologists provided will depend upon the case load.

3. Audiologist

Each center should have on its staff a Senior Audiologist who holds an Advanced Certificate in Hearing or its equivalent issued by the American Speech and Hearing Association.

4. Hearing and Speech Therapists

The hearing and speech therapists should meet the requirements for the Basic Certificate in Hearing and/or Speech issued by the American Hearing and Speech Association.

5. Psychologist

Two years' experience. Master's degree in clinical psychology. Prior experience in working with children is desirable.

6. Medical Social Worker

Should be a graduate of an accredited school of social work with two years of experience in a medical setting.

7. Nurse

A Registered Professional Nurse licensed in the State of New York, preferably with experience in working with children. Public Health Nursing experience or education is desirable.

INDEX